Ayoub El Maazouzi
Keltoum Khallouq

Educational evaluation

AF537246

Ayoub El Maazouzi
Keltoum Khallouq

Educational evaluation

Introduction

ScienciaScripts

Imprint
Any brand names and product names mentioned in this book are subject to trademark, brand or patent protection and are trademarks or registered trademarks of their respective holders. The use of brand names, product names, common names, trade names, product descriptions etc. even without a particular marking in this work is in no way to be construed to mean that such names may be regarded as unrestricted in respect of trademark and brand protection legislation and could thus be used by anyone.

Cover image: www.ingimage.com

This book is a translation from the original published under ISBN 978-620-6-72937-2.

Publisher:
Sciencia Scripts
is a trademark of
Dodo Books Indian Ocean Ltd. and OmniScriptum S.R.L publishing group

120 High Road, East Finchley, London, N2 9ED, United Kingdom
Str. Armeneasca 28/1, office 1, Chisinau MD-2012, Republic of Moldova, Europe
Managing Directors: Ieva Konstantinova, Victoria Ursu
info@omniscriptum.com

Printed at: see last page
ISBN: 978-620-8-37867-7

Table of contents

General introduction

Assessment is a fundamental part of the educational process, as it mirrors the successes and challenges encountered by students throughout their learning journey. As a measurement tool, it goes far beyond the simple awarding of marks; it plays a crucial role in understanding educational needs, identifying gaps and valuing acquired skills. In an ever-changing world, where knowledge and skills are constantly being redefined, it is imperative that assessment practices evolve too. This book is an essential resource for teachers, trainers and educational decision-makers wishing to navigate this complex and dynamic universe.

The main aim of this book is to provide an in-depth reflection on the different dimensions of evaluation in education, while proposing practical and innovative approaches. Each chapter addresses key themes, from the definitions and objectives of assessment to the tools and methods available, and the issues of inclusivity and equity. Highlighting current challenges, such as assessment in a digital context, this book also offers a forward-looking vision of the emerging trends that will shape assessment in the future.

Throughout these pages, readers will discover that assessment is not an end in itself, but rather a dynamic process that needs to be thoughtfully integrated into everyday teaching. Indeed, effective assessment must not only measure acquired knowledge, but also encourage student motivation and commitment. Assessment practices must be designed to foster active learning, where students are not only receivers of knowledge, but also actors in their own learning. In this way, this book promotes the idea that formative assessment, for example, can transform the educational journey of students, encouraging them to reflect on their learning and to assess themselves constructively.

Particular attention is also paid to inclusive assessment, essential in an educational context where student diversity is increasingly recognized. This book explores practical strategies for adapting assessment tools to students' specific needs, ensuring that everyone can participate fully in the learning process. Inclusiveness should not be seen as a mere add-on, but as a fundamental principle that enriches the entire educational experience.

Technological advances are also playing a major role in the evolution of assessment practices. In this book, we discuss digital tools that not only facilitate the implementation of varied and engaging assessments, but also offer data analysis possibilities for adjusting pedagogical strategies. Online assessment, with its advantages and challenges, is a must-read for educators wishing to adapt to contemporary demands.

This book is designed to be a practical and accessible resource, rich in concrete examples, case studies and recommendations. Both novice and experienced teachers will find tools and strategies they can easily integrate into their practice. By fostering a collaborative and reflective approach, this book aims to encourage ongoing dialogue between practitioners, researchers and trainers, with a view to evolving conceptions of assessment.

In short, this book is not just a compilation of theories and practices; it's an invitation to rethink assessment as a powerful lever for learning. It highlights the importance of thoughtful, learner-centered assessment that values skills, stimulates motivation and prepares students to meet the challenges of an ever-changing world. Whether in a traditional classroom or a digital learning environment, this book offers keys to transforming assessment into an enriching process for both students and teachers. By integrating these thoughts and practices, we have the opportunity to contribute to a more equitable, effective and inspiring educational future.

Chapter 1: Introduction, Types and Methods of Valuation

1.1 Introduction to evaluation in education

Assessment in education is a fundamental process that plays a crucial role in students' educational careers. It is not limited simply to the measurement of acquired knowledge, but also encompasses a range of objectives and functions designed to support learning and improve teaching. In this first chapter, we will explore the essential notions of assessment, starting with its definition, which will serve as a framework for understanding the different approaches and methods of assessment. We will then look at the aims of assessment, which go beyond simple grading to include coaching and the development of students' skills. Finally, we highlight the importance of assessment in the educational process, emphasizing its role as a feedback and motivational tool, as well as its impact on the quality of teaching and learning. This chapter thus lays the groundwork for understanding the issues and challenges associated with assessment in today's educational context.

1.1.1 Definition of evaluation

Assessment is a fundamental process in education, playing a key role in the development and learning of students. At its simplest, assessment can be described as a set of methods and practices for collecting, analyzing and interpreting information about the performance of an individual or group of individuals. However, such a definition, while pertinent, does not capture all the complexity and richness of this process.

Assessment goes beyond simply measuring knowledge acquired; it involves a series of actions that enable educators to understand how students learn, what they have mastered and what difficulties they encounter. In this sense, assessment is often seen as a mirror reflecting not only students' skills, but also the effectiveness of the pedagogical methods used [1].

There are a number of dimensions to valuation that are worth examining [2]. Firstly, we can distinguish between formative and summative assessment. Formative assessment takes place throughout the learning process and aims to provide continuous feedback to students. This enables them to understand their mistakes and adjust their approach before reaching a final assessment. Summative assessment, on the other hand, is carried out at the end of a learning cycle, generally to determine whether learning objectives have been achieved. These two types of assessment are complementary and play a crucial role in a student's educational journey [3].

Assessment can also be seen in terms of the different tools and methods it uses. These range from written and oral tests, to practical projects, classroom observations and self-evaluation. Each of these tools has its own strengths and weaknesses, and can be used to measure different aspects of learning. For example, tests can provide quantitative data on knowledge, while projects can offer a more qualitative view of students' ability to apply their skills in real-life situations.

Another essential dimension of assessment is its role in motivating students. By providing constructive feedback and recognizing success, assessment can stimulate students' engagement in their learning. [4]. Conversely, poorly designed assessment can lead to demotivation, excessive stress and an aversion to learning. It is therefore crucial that educators adopt a thoughtful approach to assessment, ensuring that it is both fair and equitable [4], [5].

Assessment is a complex, multi-dimensional process that plays a crucial role in education. It enables teachers to measure student progress, adapt their teaching and encourage meaningful learning. [6], [7]. To be effective, assessment must be designed to meet the diverse needs of students, while fostering a culture of learning and continuous improvement. By recognizing the richness of assessment and strategically integrating it into the educational process, teachers can truly enrich the learning experience and prepare students to succeed in a constantly changing world.

1.1.2 Assessment objectives

Assessment plays a central role in the educational process, and its objectives are many and varied. Indeed, effective assessment goes far beyond simply measuring student performance; it is a fundamental tool for improving learning, guiding teaching and fostering students' personal development. With this in mind, it is essential to understand the main objectives of assessment in order to maximize its impact on the education system.

a) **Measuring student learning:** One of the primary aims of assessment is to measure student learning. This enables us to determine the extent to which students have assimilated the knowledge and skills they have been taught. Through various assessment tools, such as tests, exams, projects or presentations, teachers can obtain precise data on student performance. This measurement is crucial, as it provides a basis for assigning grades and certifying students' skills, while identifying areas where improvement is needed [3], [8], [9]

b) **Providing constructive feedback:** Another essential aim of assessment is to provide constructive feedback to students. Feedback plays a crucial role in the learning process, enabling students to understand their strengths and weaknesses. Quality feedback, which highlights successes while suggesting areas for improvement, helps students to set clear learning goals and develop a proactive attitude towards their education. What's more, regular feedback enables students to track their progress over time, boosting their motivation and commitment.

c) **Adapting teaching :** Assessment also enables teachers to adapt their teaching methods according to students' needs [10]. By analyzing assessment results, teachers can identify gaps in learning and adjust their practices accordingly [11]. For example, if a significant number of students fail to master a particular concept, the teacher may choose to revisit that concept, explore alternative approaches or introduce complementary activities to reinforce understanding. This ability to adapt is essential to meet the diverse needs of students in the classroom [12].

d) **Informing educational decisions:** Beyond the classroom setting, assessment results provide valuable information that can influence educational decisions at an institutional level. [13]. The data collected can help schools and education systems assess the effectiveness of teaching programs and make informed decisions about curriculum development, resource allocation and teacher training [14]. Systematic, well-designed evaluation can thus play a key role in the overall improvement of educational quality [14], [15].

e) **Encouraging self-regulation and responsibility:** Assessment also aims to promote self-regulation in students [16]. By providing them with self-assessment tools and opportunities to reflect on their learning, students can develop self-regulation skills that will help them throughout their lives. [17]. By becoming aware of their own progress, challenges and learning strategies, students become more autonomous and responsible for their education. [18]. This ability to evaluate their own work is a valuable skill, not only academically, but also in other areas of life. [19].

f) **Fostering a culture of continuous learning:** Finally, a fundamental aim of assessment is to foster a culture of continuous learning. By instituting a regular and meaningful assessment practice, teachers can encourage students to perceive learning as a dynamic, ongoing process rather than a static end result. [3], [20]. Such a culture encourages students to engage in long-term learning, where curiosity, exploration and reflection are valued. It can also encourage a positive school climate, where mistakes are seen as learning opportunities rather than failures [21].

the aims of assessment in education are varied and interconnected. By measuring student achievement, providing constructive feedback, adapting teaching, informing educational decisions, encouraging self-regulation and fostering a culture of continuous learning, assessment proves to be a powerful tool in the service of education. To be effective, it must be well designed and aligned with learning objectives, ensuring that every student has the opportunity to succeed and thrive in their educational journey [4]. By integrating these objectives into daily practice, teachers can transform assessment into an essential lever for student learning and development [22].

1.1.3 The importance of evaluation in the educational process

Assessment plays a fundamental role in the educational process, acting as an essential catalyst for learning and teaching. It goes beyond simple grading and presents itself as a strategic tool that enables teachers to measure student understanding, identify gaps and guide pedagogical decisions [6]. By providing accurate data on students' skill levels, assessment helps to adjust teaching methods and personalize pedagogical approaches to meet learners' specific needs [23].

A key aspect of the importance of assessment is its ability to motivate students. When carried out constructively, assessment can encourage students to become more engaged in their learning. By providing regular, relevant feedback, teachers help students become aware of their progress and understand that learning is a continuous process. This feedback, which highlights both successes and areas for improvement, creates an environment conducive to active learning, where students feel valued and supported [4], [24], [25].

What's more, assessment is a powerful diagnostic tool. It enables teachers to identify not only students' strengths, but also their specific difficulties. Through diagnostic assessments, teachers can gain valuable information about students' prior skills, enabling them to target the interventions needed to help each student progress [26]. This preventive approach is crucial to prevent deficiencies from becoming major obstacles to future learning [27].

Assessment also plays a key role in empowering students. By taking part in assessment processes, students learn to evaluate themselves, reflect on their performance and set learning goals. [28]. This awareness encourages them to become autonomous learners, capable of regulating their own learning process. What's more, when students are involved in assessment, they develop a deeper understanding of what is expected of them, which helps them navigate their educational journey [29].

Another essential aspect is the way in which assessment informs teaching practices. Assessment results enable teachers to reflect on the effectiveness of their teaching methods and modify their approach in line with students' needs [30]. This dynamic of continuous improvement contributes not only to the development of students, but also to the professionalization of teachers, who learn to adapt their strategies according to the results obtained.

Assessment also fosters communication between teachers, students and parents. An open dialogue on assessment results creates a learning community in which each player has a role to play. [31], [32]. By being informed of their children's progress, parents can also support their children's learning at home. This collaboration between teachers and parents is crucial to creating a coherent and stimulating educational environment.

Assessment is also essential for ensuring the quality of educational programs. By collecting and analyzing data on student performance, schools can assess the effectiveness of their curricula and teaching methods. [33]. This enables educational leaders to make informed decisions about improvements to curricula and teaching resources.

In an ever-changing educational context, assessment must also evolve. The integration of technology into the assessment process offers new possibilities for measuring and monitoring student progress. Digital tools enable more efficient data collection and real-time feedback, making assessment more accessible and dynamic [34], [35]. However, it is crucial that teachers are trained to use these tools thoughtfully, to ensure that assessment remains a learner-centered process.

Finally, the importance of assessment lies in its ability to prepare students for their future. By developing skills such as critical thinking, problem-solving and collaboration through a variety of assessments, students are better equipped to navigate a complex and changing world. Assessment not only measures what has been learned, but plays a central role in the development of essential skills for students' personal and professional lives.

1.2 Types of evaluation

In today's educational landscape, evaluation is an essential process that takes a variety of forms and serves a variety of purposes. This chapter is dedicated to exploring the main types of assessment, each with its own distinct characteristics, methods and purposes. We begin by discussing formative assessment, a valuable tool for guiding learning in the process, enabling teachers and students to adjust their practices in real time. Next, we'll look at summative assessment, often used at the end of a learning cycle to measure students' achievements. We'll also look at diagnostic assessment, which aims to identify students' strengths and weaknesses before they embark on new learning, so that teaching can be better adapted. Finally, we'll look at the distinctions between normative and criterion-referenced assessment, each of which has important implications for how student results are interpreted and used. By examining these different types of assessment, this chapter aims to provide teachers and trainers with the tools and knowledge to choose the most appropriate methods according to learning contexts and objectives.

1.2.1 Diagnostic evaluation

Diagnostic assessment plays a fundamental role in the educational process, providing an in-depth understanding of students' prior knowledge, skills and specific needs before the start of a new course or learning unit. Unlike other forms of assessment, which focus on student performance at the end of a learning period, diagnostic assessment is carried out upstream and is used to inform pedagogical decisions [36].

It allows teachers to gain insight into students' strengths and weaknesses, which is crucial for tailoring instruction to individual needs [26], [37]. For example, if a diagnostic assessment reveals that a student has significant shortcomings in mathematics, the teacher may choose to differentiate his or her teaching methods to provide extra support for this student, offering remedial activities or targeted exercises that reinforce basic skills.

Diagnostic assessment can take a variety of forms, including questionnaires, tests, interviews or observations. Questionnaires can include multiple-choice questions, short answers or open-ended problems that allow students to express their understanding. Diagnostic tests are often designed to assess specific areas, such as reading comprehension or mathematical skills [38]and can be adapted to the student's grade level. Interviews also offer a valuable opportunity to understand students' perceptions of their own skills and previous learning experiences. Finally, classroom observation can provide contextual information on student behavior, motivation and engagement, enriching the data obtained by other means.

One of the main advantages of diagnostic assessment is that it enables a proactive approach to teaching. Instead of waiting for students to encounter difficulties in their learning, teachers can anticipate potential obstacles and adjust their planning accordingly. This can help create a more inclusive learning environment, where every student receives the attention and support they need to succeed. For example, in a science class, if diagnostic assessment indicates that several students are struggling with basic chemistry concepts, the teacher may decide to review these concepts before introducing more complex ideas, thus ensuring that all students have the necessary grounding to follow the program [26], [39].

In addition, diagnostic assessment fosters a culture of student-centered learning. Involving students in the assessment process gives them the opportunity to reflect on their own learning and become aware of their strengths and weaknesses. This can also boost motivation, as students feel more responsible for their own learning. Teachers can encourage this reflection by asking students to set personal learning goals based on the results of the diagnostic assessment, thus encouraging them to actively engage in their learning process [40].

However, for diagnostic assessment to be truly effective, it must be well designed and implemented. Teachers must ensure that the assessment tools used are valid and reliable, capable of accurately measuring the skills and knowledge they are intended to assess. It is also important to interpret results cautiously and to take into account the context of each student [40]. Factors such as stress, personal problems or cultural background can influence student performance in an assessment, and teachers need to be aware of these when analyzing results.

Furthermore, diagnostic assessment should not be seen as a mere administrative formality. On the contrary, it should be integrated into the classroom learning culture. Teachers can use it regularly to fine-tune their teaching throughout the school year. The results of diagnostic assessments should also be shared with students and their parents. By communicating these results, teachers can establish a partnership with parents to support students' learning at home.

Diagnostic assessment stands out not only for its knowledge assessment function, but also for its potential to establish positive relationships between teachers and students. By showing students that their progress is taken into account and that their needs are a priority, teachers foster a climate of trust and mutual respect. This can encourage open communication where students feel comfortable asking for help and sharing their concerns.

In short, diagnostic assessment is an indispensable tool in a teacher's teaching arsenal. Not only does it help to identify students' skills and prior knowledge, it also enables them to create adapted and inclusive teaching strategies. By integrating diagnostic assessments throughout the school year, teachers can provide ongoing support to students, helping them develop the skills they need to succeed in their studies.

1.2.2 Formative evaluation

Formative assessment is an essential process that accompanies student learning throughout their educational journey. Unlike summative assessment, which focuses on measuring knowledge at the end of a teaching period, formative assessment takes place on an ongoing basis, enabling teachers to gather information about students' progress as they learn. This type of assessment aims to identify students' needs, adjust teaching strategies and provide immediate, constructive feedback, thus promoting continuous improvement [41], [42].

One of the main aims of formative assessment is to create a learning environment in which students feel supported and encouraged. By incorporating regular and varied assessments, teachers can better understand students' strengths and difficulties. For example, quick quizzes, class discussions, group observations or self-assessments enable teachers to gather valuable data on students' level of understanding. This information can then be used to tailor teaching to individual needs, by offering additional resources or modifying teaching methods [41].

Another important dimension of formative evaluation is feedback. Effective feedback is specific, descriptive and action-oriented [43], [44]. It should aim to help students understand what they have done well and where they can improve. For example, instead of simply giving a grade to a piece of work, a teacher can provide feedback on the student's strengths and concrete suggestions for progress. This approach encourages students to become aware of their learning process and develop self-regulation skills, enabling them to become more autonomous learners [45].

Formative assessment also encourages collaboration between students. By incorporating peer assessment activities, teachers foster a learning climate where students can share ideas, constructively critique each other's work and learn together [46]. This type of assessment not only strengthens students' social skills, but also enables them to better understand the content by explaining their ideas to their peers.

Technology is also playing an increasingly important role in formative assessment. Digital tools, such as online assessment applications, enable teachers to quickly collect data on student performance and provide instant feedback. What's more, these platforms can offer detailed analyses of student progress, helping teachers to identify trends and adapt their teaching accordingly [47]. The use of technology also facilitates pedagogical differentiation, enabling teachers to offer activities tailored to each student's level and pace of learning [48].

Finally, integrating effective formative assessment into teaching requires adequate teacher training. They must be trained not only to design relevant assessments, but also to interpret the data collected and implement pedagogical changes based on this information. Educational establishments need to promote a culture of continuous assessment, where teachers collaborate and exchange best practices to improve the effectiveness of their assessments.

As a dynamic learning tool, formative assessment offers a multitude of benefits that enrich the educational process. By focusing on support, collaboration and feedback, it helps to create an inclusive and stimulating learning environment, where every student has the opportunity to succeed and develop to the full.

1.2.3 Summative evaluation

Summative assessment is a crucial component of the educational process, playing a decisive role in measuring students' acquisition of skills and knowledge at the end of a learning period. It usually takes place at the end of a course, semester or unit of study, providing an overall picture of student performance [49], [50]. Unlike formative assessment, which aims to support ongoing learning, the main purpose of summative assessment is to judge the effectiveness of the teaching provided and students' understanding in relation to established learning objectives.

One of the main advantages of summative assessment is that it allows learning outcomes to be quantified and student performance to be compared against specific criteria. This often translates into grades or certificates that reflect the level of competence achieved by each student. For example, in a mathematics class, a final exam may measure students' understanding of algebraic concepts, while a science project may assess their ability to apply scientific methods to a given problem. The results of these assessments can be used to rank students, award diplomas, or determine their admission to advanced or specialized programs.

Summative assessment is often criticized for its focus on the outcome rather than the learning process. However, it can be designed to reflect meaningful learning [51]. For example, by incorporating open-ended questions or projects, summative assessment can encourage students to demonstrate their understanding creatively and analytically. In addition, transparent assessment criteria enable students to understand what is expected of them and to prepare appropriately. By clearly defining learning objectives and providing a detailed assessment scale, teachers can help students focus on the skills they need to develop.

Another dimension of summative evaluation is its role in providing feedback to teachers. The results of summative assessments can provide valuable information on the effectiveness of teaching methods and curricula. By analyzing assessment data, teachers can identify trends, such as areas where students have been particularly successful or where they have encountered difficulties [52]. This can lead to a review of pedagogical practices and continuous improvement of educational programs. For example, if a large number of students fail an exam on a certain subject, this may signal a need to adjust the teaching method or provide additional support [50].

Summative assessment must also take into account the diversity of students and their specific needs. Assessments must be accessible and fair to all, taking into account cultural, linguistic and socio-economic differences. Teachers can use adaptations, such as oral tests or alternative formats, to ensure that every student has the opportunity to demonstrate their skills in a fair way. This inclusive approach is essential to ensure that all students, including those with special needs, are able to succeed within the education system.

Finally, summative assessment is a motivational tool for students [53]. It can create an opportunity for students to measure themselves against standards and achieve goals, which can strengthen their commitment and determination to learn. Well-designed assessments that incorporate elements of choice or creativity can transform this experience into a learning opportunity, rather than just a stressful moment. By incorporating aspects that value effort and progress, teachers can create an environment in which students feel encouraged to excel.

In short, summative assessment is an essential part of the educational framework, providing both information on student learning and feedback on the effectiveness of teaching practices. By designing it thoughtfully and inclusively, teachers can take advantage of its benefits while minimizing its limitations. This type of assessment, when used in conjunction with other forms of evaluation, helps to create a balanced and effective education system, capable of meeting the diverse needs of all students.

1.2.4 Normative and criterion-referenced evaluation

Normative assessment and criterion-referenced assessment are two complementary approaches that play a crucial role in the student assessment process, but they differ fundamentally in their aims and implementation. Normative assessment [54]is designed to compare the performance of students with each other within a group. This method makes it possible to situate a student in relation to his or her peers [55]using standardized statistics and measurements. For example, standardized tests are often used in normative assessments, where results are interpreted according to the score distribution of a reference group. A student with an above-average score is considered to have outperformed his or her peers, while a lower score may indicate a need for improvement.

One of the main advantages of normative assessment is its ability to identify students at the top and bottom of the performance scale. This can be particularly useful in contexts where it is important to select students for advanced programs, or to identify those who require additional support. However, this approach also has its drawbacks. By focusing primarily on comparison between students, it can encourage a competitive mentality rather than genuine learning. Furthermore, results may not accurately reflect individual understanding or skills, as they are influenced by overall group performance.

In contrast, criterion-referenced assessment focuses on measuring student performance against specific criteria or standards, independently of the performance of others [56]. This approach aims to determine the extent to which a student has achieved predefined learning objectives. For example, a test that assesses understanding of a particular concept or application of a skill will be designed with clear criteria, such as the minimum knowledge that each student must demonstrate to be considered successful. The results of criterion-referenced assessment are often expressed in terms of percentages or levels of mastery, making it possible to determine exactly which students have met, exceeded or failed to meet learning objectives.

One of the main advantages of criterion-referenced assessment is that it provides more precise and specific feedback on student performance. Based on defined criteria, this method enables teachers to identify the areas in which a student excels and those in which he or she needs improvement. It also helps create a learning environment focused on individual progress, as students can concentrate on acquiring specific skills rather than comparing themselves to their peers.

However, this approach is not without its challenges. To be effective, criterion-referenced assessment requires well-defined and clear criteria, which can require considerable work on the part of teachers to ensure that these criteria are relevant and appropriate for all students [57]. In addition, results can be influenced by external factors, such as socio-economic background, which can affect students' ability to achieve these criteria.

In practice, many educators integrate the two approaches to offer a more complete and balanced assessment. By using both normative and criterion-referenced assessment, teachers can benefit from the strengths of each method while minimizing their respective weaknesses. For example, normative assessment can be used to identify general trends within a group of students, while criterion-referenced assessment can provide detailed information on the specific skills each student needs to develop.

Combining the two approaches can also help develop targeted intervention strategies for students. By identifying both above- and below-average students in a normative assessment, and using clear criteria to understand each student's performance, teachers can better target their efforts to meet the diverse needs of their students.

In short, normative assessment and criterion-referenced assessment are two essential approaches which, when used in a complementary way, offer a more complete picture of student performance. When used together, they provide an in-depth understanding of students' strengths and weaknesses, promoting more effective learning tailored to each student's individual needs.

Conclusion

Assessment in education is a multidimensional and essential process that goes far beyond the simple measurement of performance. It enriches the learning experience, encourages student engagement, and contributes to their academic, personal and social development. The diversity of types of assessment - formative, summative, diagnostic, normative and criterion-referenced - testifies to the complexity and richness of this process. Each type of assessment plays a specific role: formative assessment provides constructive feedback for ongoing adjustment, while summative assessment measures final achievements. Diagnostic assessment, on the other hand, identifies needs for personalized learning.

By recognizing these complementary approaches, teachers can design assessment strategies that are adapted to students' varied pedagogical objectives and needs, thus creating an inclusive and equitable educational culture. Faced with the challenges of an ever-changing world, it becomes crucial to adopt innovative assessment practices that prepare students for their future role as citizens. This chapter lays the foundations for an in-depth reflection on assessment methods and approaches, paving the way for practical explorations in the following chapters.

Chapter 2: Designing and implementing an assessment system

2.1 Assessment tools and methods

Assessment in the field of education does not rely solely on quantitative instruments, but encompasses a variety of tools and methods that provide a comprehensive view of students' skills and knowledge. This chapter focuses on the main assessment tools and methods used in the educational process. We begin with an analysis of tests and examinations, which remain common practice for measuring student learning in a standardized way. Next, we'll explore projects and assignments, which foster a more active and engaging approach to learning, enabling students to demonstrate their skills in a creative and concrete way. We'll also look at classroom observations, a valuable tool for assessing student behaviors and interactions in a real learning context. Finally, we'll look at peer and self-assessment, methods that encourage critical thinking and autonomy in students' learning processes. Through this exploration, this chapter aims to provide teachers with an in-depth understanding of different assessment tools and methods, as well as strategies for effectively integrating them into their daily practice.

2.1.1 Tests and examinations

Tests and examinations are widely used assessment tools in education, enabling the acquisition of students' knowledge and skills to be measured in a structured, standardized way. These instruments play an essential role in summative assessment, providing teachers and institutions with a clear view of students' understanding at the end of a learning period, module or entire course.

Tests can take many forms, from multiple-choice questionnaires to open-ended questions and practical exercises. Multiple-choice tests are often preferred for their ease of administration and evaluation. They enable rapid correction and offer quantifiable results that can be analyzed statistically. However, although these tests can cover a wide range of knowledge, they are sometimes criticized for their limited ability to assess students' critical thinking and deep understanding.

On the other hand, open-ended questions and written tests offer greater scope for expressing complex ideas, analysis and reasoning. These formats encourage students to think critically and demonstrate their understanding through written expression. Nevertheless, the assessment of these responses can be more subjective, requiring clear scales and well-defined evaluation criteria to ensure a fair appraisal of performance.

Examinations, which are often longer and more comprehensive than tests, generally encompass a variety of question formats, from MCQs to essays. They are often used at the end of a school year or study cycle to assess the overall knowledge acquired. Examinations can also include practical components, particularly in subjects such as science or the arts, where students are required to demonstrate specific skills in real or simulated situations.

One of the main advantages of tests and examinations is their ability to provide objective, quantifiable data on student performance. [58]. This enables teachers to identify the areas in which students excel and those in which they struggle. By analyzing the results, teachers can adjust their teaching methods and offer targeted support to students in difficulty, thus promoting more effective learning.

However, the use of tests and exams also brings its own challenges. One of the main risks is the pressure they put on students. Fear of failure and exam anxiety can affect students' performance, preventing them from giving their best. This can also lead to intensive preparation practices, focusing on memorization rather than actual understanding of concepts. In this context, it is essential that teachers create a positive assessment environment that values learning and encourages students to take a proactive approach to testing.

The design of tests and exams must also be carefully thought through to ensure that they actually measure what they are intended to assess. Teachers need to ensure that questions are clear, relevant and aligned with learning objectives. A good test should cover a range of difficulty levels, allowing basic knowledge to be assessed while challenging students to demonstrate more advanced skills.

In addition, it is crucial to take into account the diversity of students when designing tests and exams. [59]. Teachers should strive to adapt assessments so that they are accessible to all, taking into account different learning styles, cultural backgrounds and special educational needs. This may include providing extra time for students with special needs, as well as alternative formats for tests.

Assessment through tests and examinations must also be integrated into a broader system of assessment, which includes other assessment methods, such as formative assessment and projects. Tests and examinations should not be the sole indicators of a student's success, but rather a complement to other forms of assessment that offer a more complete picture of students' skills and knowledge.

Finally, the results of tests and examinations can provide valuable information for parents, students and educational institutions. They can form the basis for decisions on student placement, curriculum and teacher professional development. By sharing these results in a transparent way, schools can also foster parental involvement in their children's educational journey. So, while tests and examinations have undeniable advantages as assessment tools, they should be used with caution and as a complement to other evaluation methods. They should be designed to encourage learning and critical thinking, rather than being seen solely as a means of measuring academic performance. By adopting a balanced and considered approach to assessment, teachers can maximize the benefits of tests and exams while minimizing their drawbacks.

2.1.2 Projects and practical work

Projects and practical work are essential pedagogical tools for student assessment, as they enable theoretical knowledge to be applied to concrete situations. By promoting active learning, these methods encourage students to become more involved in their learning process. Projects offer an opportunity to explore subjects in depth, while practical work helps to develop specific technical and practical skills [60], [61].

When designing projects and assignments, it's crucial to establish clear, measurable learning objectives. These objectives guide students through the process and help them understand what is expected of them. For example, a project on conducting a scientific experiment might aim to have students learn how to formulate hypotheses, design experiments, collect and analyze data, and communicate their results. By defining precise objectives, teachers can better assess the skills acquired by students.

Group projects are particularly beneficial, as they foster collaboration and teamwork [62]. In a professional world increasingly focused on teamwork, these interpersonal skills are essential. By working together, students learn to share responsibilities, negotiate ideas and resolve conflicts. Teachers can incorporate elements of collaborative assessment, where each member of the group is accountable for his or her contribution, enabling a fairer evaluation of the collective effort.

Integrating technology into projects and assignments can also enrich the learning experience. For example, students can use simulation software to model scientific concepts, or create digital presentations to share their findings. The use of technology not only stimulates student engagement, but also enables them to acquire essential digital skills in the modern world.

Another dimension of projects and practical work is the possibility of peer assessment. This method enables students to give and receive constructive feedback on their work. By engaging in critical reflection, students develop their ability to assess the quality of others' work, while receiving different perspectives on their own project. This process reinforces their understanding of evaluation criteria and motivates them to improve their performance.

Projects and practical work also offer a wide variety of assessment approaches. Instead of limiting themselves to written tests, teachers can assess students on the basis of the creativity, originality and rigor of their work. This enables a more holistic assessment of students' skills, taking into account not only the knowledge they have acquired, but also their ability to think critically and solve problems.

It's essential that teachers provide constructive feedback on students' projects and practical work. Regular feedback helps students understand where they excel and where they can improve. It also gives them an opportunity to reflect on their learning process, so that they can identify their strengths and weaknesses. Establishing an open dialogue between teacher and student is essential, enabling students to ask questions and deepen their understanding of the concepts covered.

A particularly important aspect of projects and practical work is the connection between academic learning and the real world. [63]. By integrating projects that deal with current issues or are related to the community, teachers help students see the relevance of what they are learning [64]. For example, a science project on renewable energies can encourage students to explore local solutions to environmental problems. This contextualized approach makes learning more meaningful and engaging.

Finally, projects and practical work enable students to develop self-regulation and time management skills. By managing a project, students learn to plan, prioritize and meet deadlines. These organizational skills are crucial to their future success, both academically and professionally.

By integrating projects and practical work into the assessment process, teachers offer an enriching and varied learning experience that prepares students to meet complex challenges in an ever-changing world.

2.1.3 Classroom observations

Classroom observation is a qualitative assessment method that enables teachers to obtain valuable information about students' behavior, engagement and interactions in a learning environment. By observing students during school activities, teachers can assess not only academic achievement, but also students' social and emotional development, which is essential for a well-rounded education.

This approach is based on the principle that learning is not just about acquiring theoretical knowledge, but also includes interpersonal skills and attitudes to learning. By observing students, teachers can identify group dynamics, individual learning styles and the specific challenges each student faces. For example, some students may excel in group activities, demonstrating strong communication and collaboration skills, while others may need more time or a quiet environment to concentrate [65], [66].

Observations can be structured or unstructured. Structured observations follow a specific protocol, where teachers use predefined observation grids to assess particular criteria, such as class participation, behavior, or peer interactions [67]. These grids collect quantitative data that can be analyzed to identify trends and patterns of behavior within the classroom. For example, a teacher might use a grid to record how often each student participates in group discussions, which can help identify students who could benefit from extra support to become more involved.

On the other hand, unstructured observations are more flexible and allow teachers to capture spontaneous moments of learning. These observations can include informal student interactions, unplanned discussions and hands-on activities. For example, during a group project, a teacher might note how students collaborate and solve problems together. This can provide insights into how students apply their knowledge in real-life situations and how they interact with their peers. Teachers can also observe non-verbal behaviors, such as facial expression and body language, which can reveal levels of engagement or understanding not always evident through standardized tests.

Another important dimension of classroom observations is teacher self-reflection. By taking the time to observe their students, teachers can also reflect on their own teaching practice. This encourages them to evaluate the effectiveness of their teaching methods and adjust their approach according to the specific needs of their class [65], [66]. For example, if a teacher notices that a group of students seems disinterested during a lesson, he or she may decide to modify the format of the activity to encourage more active participation.

Classroom observations are also essential for pedagogical differentiation. By carefully observing students, teachers can identify diverse learning styles and individual needs, enabling them to adapt their teaching accordingly [68]. For example, a student who struggles with abstract concepts may benefit from hands-on activities that make learning more tangible. By incorporating these observations into their practice, teachers can create an inclusive learning environment where every student has the opportunity to succeed.

It is also important to establish an ethical framework for classroom observations. Teachers need to ensure that students are aware that they are being observed, and that observations are used to enhance learning, not to punish. Open communication with students about the observation process fosters a climate of trust and security, enabling students to feel comfortable and confident to participate fully.

Observations can also be enriched by collaboration with other teachers. By working together, teachers can share their observations and reflections, which can lead to improved teaching practices. For example, teams of teachers can observe lessons taught by colleagues to gather different perspectives and exchange ideas on effective teaching strategies.

Classroom observations can be documented in a number of ways, including written notes, video or audio recordings, or even logbooks. These documents can serve as a valuable reference for teachers when assessing student progress over time. By keeping a record of observations, teachers can track changes in student behavior and engagement, as well as the effectiveness of interventions put in place.

It's crucial that teachers integrate the results of their observations into their instructional planning. Using the data collected during observations, teachers can design lessons and activities that meet the identified needs of their students. This promotes more personalized and relevant learning, ensuring that each student receives the support they need to achieve their learning goals. In short, classroom observations are a powerful tool for enriching the learning experience for both students and teachers, and are an essential component of holistic and effective assessment.

2.1.4 Peer and self-assessment

Peer and self-assessment are pedagogical approaches that encourage students to actively engage in their own and their peers' learning. These assessment practices, which are increasingly recognized for their potential to enrich the educational experience, enable students to develop critical, analytical and reflective skills [69].

Peer assessment involves students examining and evaluating the work of their peers according to established criteria. This process encourages a culture of collaboration and dialogue between students, fostering mutual learning. By assessing the work of others, students are encouraged to analyze assessment criteria in depth, provide constructive feedback and reflect on their own work by comparing it with that of their peers [70]. This approach helps to reinforce their understanding of expectations and quality standards. In addition, giving feedback to their peers can increase their self-confidence and motivation, as they realize that their opinions and assessments are valued.

Self-assessment, on the other hand, involves students reflecting on their own learning and evaluating their performance against defined criteria. This practice encourages autonomy and responsibility, enabling students to become aware of their strengths and weaknesses. By self-assessing, students develop self-regulation skills, enabling them to better manage their learning and identify realistic goals for their progress. Self-assessment also fosters metacognition, i.e. students' ability to reflect on their own learning process, understand how they learn best and adjust their strategies accordingly.

The implementation of peer and self-assessment requires adequate preparation on the part of teachers. It is essential to clearly explain assessment criteria and provide concrete examples so that students understand what is expected of them. Teachers also need to establish a positive and respectful classroom environment, where students feel comfortable giving and receiving feedback. Class discussions on the importance of peer and self-assessment can also help emphasize their value in the learning process.

Another important dimension is training students in evaluation. This can include workshops or training sessions where students learn how to formulate constructive comments, how to analyze work according to evaluation criteria, and how to use evaluation grids. By providing them with tools and strategies for carrying out these assessments, teachers help them to become competent assessors, able to reflect critically on their own learning and that of others.

Peer and self-assessment also have a significant impact on student motivation. By actively participating in the assessment process, students feel more involved in their learning. This can increase their interest in the subject and their commitment to school activities. The opportunity to assess the work of others and see their own progress can boost their self-esteem and confidence in their abilities.

However, these evaluation methods are not without their challenges. Teachers need to be aware of potential biases that can influence peer assessments, such as friendships or rivalries. It is important to develop mechanisms to mitigate these biases, such as anonymous rubrics or peers who are not directly related to the student being assessed. In addition, teachers need to ensure that self-evaluation is sincere and thoughtful. This may require coaching and regular discussions on how to assess one's own work objectively.

By integrating peer and self-assessment into the pedagogical framework, teachers foster active, participatory learning. These practices enable students to become active players in their own education, developing essential skills for their academic and professional future. The use of these methods also contributes to the creation of a dynamic learning community, where students help and encourage each other on their educational journey.

2.2: Designing an evaluation system

The design of an evaluation system is a strategic process of paramount importance in ensuring the coherence and effectiveness of evaluative practices in the educational field. This chapter explores the fundamental elements underlying the design of such a system. We begin by examining the principles of evaluation design, which form the foundation on which all evaluation methods and tools are built. These principles guide educators in creating assessments that are relevant and adapted to students' needs, while taking into account diverse learning contexts. Next, we'll look at the alignment of learning objectives with assessments, an essential aspect in ensuring that assessment tools truly measure the skills and knowledge targeted by the program. Finally, we'll discuss success criteria and scales, which are crucial to providing clear and accurate feedback to students, enabling them to understand their performance and actively engage in their learning. Through this exploration, this chapter aims to provide teachers with the necessary foundations to design an effective assessment system, capable of fostering learning and improving educational outcomes.

2.2.1 Assessment design principles

The design of an assessment system is based on several fundamental principles that guarantee its effectiveness and relevance. These principles guide educators' decisions about how to measure student learning, collect data and use the results to improve teaching and learning. [71].

One of the first principles of evaluation design is clarity of purpose. It is crucial that learning objectives are clearly defined and understood by all those involved. These objectives must be specific, measurable, achievable, realistic and time-bound (SMART). [72]. By establishing clear objectives, teachers can align assessment methods with expected learning outcomes, making it easier to measure student progress. Students, for their part, know what is expected of them, enabling them to better prepare for assessments [73].

Another important principle is validity. Validity refers to the ability of an assessment to measure what it is intended to measure. To ensure validity, it is essential to choose assessment tools that correspond to the learning objectives [74], [75]. For example, if the aim is to measure students' ability to apply theoretical concepts in practical situations, it would be inappropriate to rely solely on a written test. Instead, an assessment based on a practical project or simulation would be more appropriate. Validity also means ensuring that the assessment is not influenced by external factors, such as stress or anxiety, which could distort the results.

Reliability is another fundamental principle of evaluation design. It refers to the consistency of assessment results when administered under similar conditions. For an assessment to be reliable, it is important that assessment criteria are applied consistently and that the tools used are precise enough to measure student performance consistently [76], [77]. This may require training for assessors to ensure a common understanding of criteria and expectations. For example, when assessing written work, detailed rubrics can help standardize the process and ensure that every student is assessed according to the same criteria.

Another key principle is equity. Assessment must be designed to ensure equal opportunities for success for all students, whatever their background, ability or special needs. This means adapting assessment tools so that they are accessible to all students, including those with special educational needs. For example, adjustments can be made for dyslexic students, such as the use of extra time or the possibility of answering questions orally. By incorporating inclusive assessment practices, teachers create an equitable learning environment that recognizes and values student diversity [78], [79].

An often overlooked but equally important principle is relevance. [80]. Assessments must be relevant to the learning context and related to students' real lives. Students are more likely to engage in the learning process when they see the value and applicability of what they are learning. Therefore, it is essential to design assessments that reflect real-world scenarios, enabling students to apply their skills in practical situations. This can include case studies, group projects or simulations that mimic real-world challenges.

Feedback is another critical aspect of evaluation design [81]. Effective assessment involves more than simply awarding a grade; it must also include constructive feedback that helps students understand their performance and identify areas for improvement. Feedback must be specific, precise and action-oriented, enabling students to know exactly what they need to do to make progress [82]. By building regular feedback mechanisms into the assessment system, teachers foster a continuous learning cycle that helps students develop self-reflective skills.

And finally, an essential principle of evaluation design is flexibility [83], [84]. Assessment systems must be adaptable to meet the changing needs of students and evolving educational contexts. Teachers must be prepared to re-evaluate and adjust their assessment methods in response to results, student feedback and changes in the curriculum. This ability to adapt ensures that assessment remains relevant and effective, even in a constantly changing educational environment.

By integrating these assessment design principles, teachers can create robust and effective assessment systems that promote student learning. These assessment systems should be viewed not only as measurement tools, but also as levers for continuous improvement in teaching and learning. By adopting a thoughtful and systematic approach to assessment design, educators are better equipped to support the development of students' skills and knowledge, thus contributing to their academic and personal success.

2.2.2 Aligning learning objectives and assessments

The alignment of learning objectives and assessments is a fundamental principle in the design of an effective assessment system. This process ensures that assessments measure precisely what students are expected to learn, providing relevant data on their progress and understanding. To achieve this alignment, it is essential to follow several key steps, each helping to ensure that assessment supports and reflects the defined learning objectives [85].

First of all, it's crucial to clearly define learning objectives. These objectives should be precisely formulated, indicating what students should know and be able to do by the end of a lesson or unit. For example, instead of saying "Students will understand photosynthesis", it's more appropriate to specify "Students will be able to explain the process of photosynthesis, using appropriate terms and describing its various stages". This formulation helps to orient the development of assessments towards measurable and observable criteria [85], [86], [87].

Once learning objectives have been established, it is essential to identify the types of assessment best suited to measure these objectives. Assessment can take many forms, including formative, summative, projects, oral presentations or exams. Each type of assessment should be chosen according to how well it measures the specific skills and knowledge related to the learning objectives.

The next step is to develop assessment criteria that reflect the learning objectives. These criteria serve as a guide for students and teachers, setting clear expectations for what constitutes successful performance. Teachers can use assessment grids to describe expected levels of performance, specifying the elements to be considered for each criterion. For example, for a science project, criteria might include accuracy of data, clarity of presentation, and ability to draw conclusions based on results. These grids help to ensure that evaluations are consistent and fair, by providing a transparent framework for assessments.

Another important dimension of alignment is taking into account the various levels of difficulty of learning objectives. Teachers must ensure that assessments are appropriate for the students' level of competence [88], [89]. For example, a learning objective may be divided into several sub-objectives, ranging from basic comprehension to more advanced skills. Assessments should reflect this progression, allowing students to demonstrate their understanding at different levels. This not only promotes student engagement, but also their motivation to achieve higher goals.

Alignment must also take into account the learning context and specific needs of the students. Every classroom is unique, with students of varying backgrounds, interests and learning styles. Teachers need to adapt their assessments so that they are relevant and accessible to all students. This can include using different assessment methods to meet diverse needs, such as oral assessment options for students who excel at verbal communication or visual assessments for those who are more art-oriented.

In addition, continuous assessment of the alignment between learning objectives and assessments is essential. This means regularly reviewing assessments to ensure that they remain aligned with learning objectives. Teachers can collect data on student performance to identify trends or gaps in learning. For example, if many students fail a test on a specific learning objective, this may indicate that the objective is not clearly understood, or that the assessment is not adequate to measure that skill. In this case, adjustments need to be made, whether by clarifying objectives, modifying assessment or providing additional support to students.

Finally, the alignment of learning objectives and assessments must also involve students in the process. When they understand the learning objectives and assessment criteria, students are more likely to be actively engaged in their learning. Teachers can encourage this participation by involving students in the creation of assessment criteria, or by allowing them to reflect on their own performance. This fosters a sense of responsibility and commitment, boosting their motivation to achieve set goals.

2.2.3 Success criteria and scales

Success criteria and scales are essential elements in the design of an assessment system [90], [91]. They enable a clear definition of what it means to succeed in a specific task or project, while providing an objective basis for assessing student performance. By establishing well-defined criteria and transparent scales, teachers foster an equitable learning culture, where every student knows what is expected and can be guided towards achieving learning goals.

Achieve to be considered as having successfully completed a task. These criteria must be precise, measurable and directly related to the learning objectives [92], [93]. If a learning goal is for students to be able to write an argumentative essay, success criteria might include clarity of thesis, logical structure of argument, quality of evidence presented and command of language. By clarifying these expectations, teachers help students understand what they need to achieve in order to succeed.

Scales, on the other hand, are tools that translate success criteria into quantifiable performance levels. A scale can be in the form of points, mastery levels or letters, and it establishes a scale for evaluating student performance in relation to defined criteria [94], [95]. For example, a four-level scale might classify performance as follows: "Excellent" for complete mastery of the criteria, "Satisfactory" for partial mastery, "Insufficient" for work that does not meet expectations, and "Not submitted" for work not handed in. Such a scale provides a nuanced assessment and helps differentiate students' skill levels.

The development of success criteria and scales requires careful thought. Teachers need to ensure that the criteria are realistic and accessible, while maintaining a high standard. This may involve collaboration with other educators to ensure that criteria are in line with academic standards and program expectations. It is also essential to involve students in the process. By consulting them on the formulation of criteria and scales, teachers foster a sense of ownership and commitment among students, which can reinforce their motivation and personal responsibility for their learning [96], [97], [98].

Success criteria and scales must also be clearly communicated to students before the start of an assessment task. This can be done through class discussions, handouts or presentations. Students must be given the opportunity to ask questions and clarify their doubts about what is expected of them [99]. By providing full transparency about the assessment criteria, teachers enable students to better prepare themselves and focus on the aspects of their work that matter most [100].

The use of evaluation grids is an effective approach for articulating success criteria and scales. [101]. An evaluation grid presents evaluation criteria on one axis, while performance levels are indicated on another axis. Each cell of the grid describes the quality of performance at that level for that criterion. For example, for a criterion concerning clarity of thesis in an essay, the grid might indicate that an "Excellent" performance presents a clear and convincing thesis, while an "Insufficient" performance presents a vague or unconvincing thesis. This approach enables teachers to provide detailed, targeted feedback to students, showing them not only where they have succeeded, but also where they can improve [102].

It's also essential to consider student diversity when designing success criteria and scales. Each student has unique strengths and weaknesses, and criteria need to be flexible to allow students to demonstrate their learning in different ways. For example, some students may excel in written tasks, while others may shine in oral presentations or practical projects. Teachers should therefore consider providing several assessment options that correspond to different learning styles and skills.

In addition, it is crucial to evaluate the effectiveness of success criteria and scales after they have been implemented. Teachers need to analyze assessment results to determine whether the criteria have been understood and applied effectively [103]. This may involve collecting feedback from students on their understanding of the criteria and the clarity of the scales used. If shortcomings are identified, adjustments should be made to improve the relevance and clarity of the criteria and scales for future assessments.

Establishing clear success criteria and transparent scales encourages constructive formative and summative assessment, where students are actively engaged in their learning. This not only measures students' performance, but also provides them with valuable feedback to guide their progress. By integrating these elements into the assessment system, teachers help to create a learning culture where every student has the opportunity to understand their performance, identify their needs for improvement and develop their skills in a meaningful and reflective way.

2.3 Assessment of skills and knowledge

The assessment of skills and knowledge represents a fundamental pillar of modern education, as it measures not only students' academic achievements, but also their ability to apply this knowledge in a variety of contexts. This chapter focuses on the different dimensions of this assessment, highlighting the various types of skills that need to be taken into account in the educational process. We begin by addressing the assessment of practical skills, which is crucial in preparing students for real-life situations where they need to mobilize their know-how. Next, we'll look at the assessment of theoretical knowledge, which remains a key element in ensuring a solid foundation on which students can build. Finally, we'll look at the assessment of cross-curricular competencies, which encompass essential skills such as critical thinking, creativity and collaboration, often crucial to success in today's world. Through this exploration, this chapter aims to provide a holistic and integrated view of the different dimensions of assessment, enabling educators to design assessment approaches that fully reflect the diversity of skills needed in contemporary society.

2.3.1 Assessment of practical skills

Assessment of practical skills is an essential component of overall student assessment, particularly in disciplines that require concrete applications of theoretical knowledge. This form of assessment measures not only what students know, but also their ability to apply this knowledge in real or simulated situations. The assessment of practical skills proves crucial in preparing students for future careers, providing them with the tools they need to succeed in professional environments that require both technical mastery and interpersonal skills [104], [105], [106].

Assessment of practical skills can take a variety of forms, from laboratory projects and simulations to live demonstrations and work placements. In the school context, laboratory projects are particularly common in science subjects, where students are required to design and carry out experiments [60], [107]. In a chemistry course, for example, students could be tasked with carrying out an experiment on acid-base reactions, and their assessment would be based not only on the results obtained, but also on their ability to follow protocols, use equipment correctly and analyze data.

Simulations are another effective way of assessing practical skills. They enable students to apply their knowledge in a controlled environment that mimics real-world situations. For example, in a management course, students could take part in a business decision-making simulation, where they have to develop strategies and solve problems as a team. This approach promotes not only the development of technical skills, but also interpersonal skills such as collaboration, communication and time management [108], [109].

Another common method of assessing practical skills is direct observation. Here, teachers can assess students as they perform specific tasks. For example, in a health sciences course, a teacher may observe students taking vital signs or performing other clinical skills. Direct observation enables teachers to gather qualitative data on student performance, assess confidence levels and identify areas for improvement. To ensure accurate and fair assessment, it is essential that teachers establish clear criteria for the skills to be assessed [110], [111], [112].

Learning portfolios are also a valuable tool for assessing practical skills. In them, students can collect evidence of their learning, including work samples, reflections on their learning process and peer assessments [113]. Portfolios enable students to demonstrate their progress over time and reflect on their learning experiences. In addition, they provide teachers with an in-depth insight into students' practical skills and their ability to self-assess their work. By encouraging students to take responsibility for their learning, portfolios help to develop skills of self-reflection and metacognition [114].

Another essential aspect of practical skills assessment is the integration of relevant assessment criteria. To ensure the validity and reliability of the assessment, it is crucial that teachers define clear criteria that reflect the specific skills to be assessed. Feedback also plays a key role in the assessment of practical skills. Constructive feedback enables students to understand their strengths and weaknesses, and to develop action plans to improve their performance. Teachers should provide specific comments, based on the assessment criteria, and suggest strategies for progress.

It's also important to recognize student diversity when assessing practical skills. Each student may have different learning styles and abilities, which means that assessment methods need to be flexible to meet these varied needs. Teachers should consider using different assessment approaches that allow each student to demonstrate their skills in an appropriate way: a student who excels at practical tasks might have the opportunity to demonstrate their skills through a concrete project, while another student might demonstrate their skills through a written presentation or group work.

assessment of practical skills should be a continuous process, enabling students to engage in an iterative learning cycle. By incorporating formative assessments throughout the year, teachers can help students identify areas for improvement and implement strategies for progress. For example, regular assessments in the form of feedback on projects or demonstrations can provide valuable insights into understanding practical skills. This encourages students to adopt a proactive attitude to their learning and seek opportunities to hone their skills.

2.3.2 Assessment of theoretical knowledge

Assessment of theoretical knowledge is an essential component of the educational process, as it measures students' understanding of concepts, ideas and theories that form the basis of their learning. Unlike the assessment of practical skills, which focuses on the concrete application of knowledge, the assessment of theoretical knowledge aims to determine the extent to which students have assimilated information, understood theories and can articulate them coherently. This form of assessment is crucial to developing a solid knowledge base on which students can build more advanced skills.

Assessments of theoretical knowledge can take many forms, including written tests, examinations, homework, oral presentations and research projects. Written tests, such as MCQs (multiple-choice questions), open-ended questions and case studies, are among the most common methods of assessing theoretical knowledge. These assessments enable teachers to check students' understanding of specific topics, assess their ability to apply their knowledge to new situations and analyze their ability to solve theoretical problems [115].

One of the advantages of written tests is that they can be administered on a large scale, making it possible to compare student performance within a class or school. However, it is essential that these tests are well designed to ensure that they actually measure conceptual understanding rather than memorization skills [116], [117]. An effective test should include questions that require students to demonstrate their understanding by explaining concepts, making connections between ideas or applying theories to practical scenarios. This ensures that the assessment reflects a thorough understanding of theoretical knowledge.

Homework and research projects also provide a valuable opportunity to assess theoretical knowledge. These assignments allow students to dive deeper into a topic, conduct research, develop arguments and synthesize information. For example, a research project on a scientific topic would enable students to explore theories and concepts in depth, examine relevant case studies and present their findings in a structured way. This approach fosters autonomy and encourages students to become active learners, helping them to integrate theoretical knowledge into a wider context.

Oral presentations are another effective way of assessing theoretical knowledge. They offer students the opportunity to present their ideas and demonstrate their understanding of concepts in front of their peers. In preparing a presentation, students are required to organize their thoughts, structure their discourse and answer questions, thus reinforcing their mastery of the subject. What's more, this method fosters the development of communication skills, essential for their academic and professional future.

The integration of assessment of theoretical knowledge within a broader framework of formative assessment is also essential. Formative assessment focuses on monitoring students' progress throughout their learning process, rather than limiting itself to one-off assessments. In addition, it is crucial to adopt a differentiated approach when assessing theoretical knowledge. Students have diverse learning styles, and it's important that assessment methods take this into account. By offering a range of assessment options, teachers can enable each student to demonstrate their understanding in the way that suits them best.

Finally, it is essential to recognize the role of motivation in the assessment of theoretical knowledge. Students who feel motivated and engaged are more likely to succeed. Teachers can stimulate student motivation by making assessments interesting and relevant, linking theoretical content to real-life situations and encouraging intellectual curiosity. For example, class discussions on topical subjects or projects that explore contemporary issues can spark students' interest and encourage them to become more involved in their learning.

2.3.3 Assessing cross-disciplinary skills

The assessment of cross-curricular skills has become an essential aspect of modern education, as it measures aptitudes and attitudes that transcend specific subjects. These skills, often referred to as "soft skills", include communication, collaboration, critical thinking, creativity, problem-solving and time management. Unlike theoretical knowledge or practical skills, which may be easier to assess using traditional methods, the assessment of cross-curricular skills requires innovative and tailored approaches [118], [119], [120], [121].

Cross-disciplinary skills are essential for students' success in a variety of contexts, both academic and professional. In a constantly evolving world, where the demands of the job market are changing rapidly, these skills play a crucial role in preparing students to adapt and succeed in a variety of environments. Employers are increasingly looking for candidates who can work as part of a team, think critically and communicate effectively. As a result, integrating the assessment of cross-curricular skills into the school curriculum has become a priority for educators.

Teachers can adopt a variety of strategies to assess cross-curricular skills. One of the most effective methods is project-based assessment. Collaborative projects enable students to work together to solve complex problems, communicate ideas and manage tasks. By observing students' interactions, their ability to share roles, meet deadlines and adjust their work in response to feedback, teachers can assess skills such as collaboration and communication. Oral presentations and debates are also effective ways of assessing cross-curricular skills. When students present a topic in front of their peers, they must not only master the content, but also communicate their ideas clearly and engagingly. In addition, debates encourage students to develop their critical thinking skills and their ability to argue logically and convincingly. [122], [123]. These activities offer teachers the opportunity to assess not only communication skills, but also students' ability to listen, respect the opinions of others and respond appropriately.

It's also important to involve students in the process of assessing cross-curricular skills. Self-assessment and peer assessment are powerful methods that enable students to reflect on their own learning and give constructive feedback to their peers. For example, after a presentation, students can evaluate each other using rubrics based on clear criteria. This helps them not only to develop critical evaluation skills, but also to understand performance expectations. What's more, this approach fosters a positive classroom climate, where students support each other in their learning.

Another essential aspect of cross-curricular skills assessment is the integration of clear, measurable learning objectives. Teachers need to define what cross-curricular competencies mean in the context of their teaching. The assessment of cross-curricular skills can also be enhanced by the use of specific assessment grids. These grids can be used to assess student performance on various criteria related to cross-curricular competencies.

It's also important to recognize that assessment of cross-curricular skills is not limited to specific moments of formal assessment. Ongoing formative assessment is essential to monitor the development of students' skills throughout the school year. For example, teachers can integrate weekly reflections on collaboration or communication into lessons, enabling students to assess their own progress. This ongoing approach encourages students to become actively engaged in their learning and aware of the importance of cross-curricular skills in their daily lives.

By integrating the assessment of cross-curricular skills into the curriculum, teachers are helping to create holistic learners, capable of navigating a complex, interconnected world. Cross-curricular skills are essential to students' success, both academically and professionally, and their appropriate assessment is crucial to ensuring that students are well prepared for the future. By adopting a varied and thoughtful approach to assessing these skills, teachers foster a learning environment that is dynamic, inclusive and focused on developing the skills needed to succeed in life.

Conclusion

Assessment in education needs to be approached holistically, integrating a diversity of tools, methods and design principles to foster rich learning adapted to the varied needs of students. Tests and examinations provide quantitative benchmarks, but it is essential to add projects, practical work and classroom observations for a more contextual and dynamic assessment. The integration of self- and peer assessment encourages individual responsibility, collaboration and critical thinking, contributing to an inclusive learning environment.

A well-designed assessment system is based on a clear alignment between learning objectives and assessment criteria, ensuring that students are assessed on what they are actually taught. The definition of explicit success criteria and scales strengthens student commitment by clarifying expectations and facilitating constructive feedback. Assessing practical skills, theoretical knowledge and cross-disciplinary competencies prepares students for the challenges of professional and social life, and promotes essential qualities such as creativity and teamwork.

In short, this chapter highlights the importance of designing diversified and balanced assessments, adapted to the demands of an ever-changing world. It paves the way for ongoing reflection on the implementation of assessment systems that enrich the learning experience and prepare students to become active, engaged citizens.

Chapter 3: Inclusive assessment

3.1: Inclusive assessment

Inclusive assessment is a fundamental concept in the modern educational framework, which aims to ensure that all students, regardless of their abilities or specific needs, have equitable access to meaningful learning opportunities. This chapter explores the practices, strategies and adaptations needed to implement inclusive assessment. We begin by examining assessment practices for students with special needs, emphasizing the importance of an individualized approach that takes into account the particularities of each student. Next, we'll look at strategies for fostering inclusion and equity in assessment, essential to creating a respectful and rewarding learning environment for all. Finally, we'll look at the adaptation of assessment tools, which plays a crucial role in measuring student learning, making it possible to respond to diverse needs and learning styles. Through this exploration, this chapter aims to provide practical guidance and reflections on how to make assessment more inclusive, thereby contributing to an education system that is more equitable and representative of learners' diversity.

3.1.1 Assessment practices for students with special needs

Assessment practices for students with special needs are essential to ensure that all students, regardless of ability, have the opportunity to succeed in their educational journey. These students may include those with learning disabilities, physical handicaps, hearing or visual impairments, and other conditions that can affect their academic performance. It is crucial that teachers adopt adapted assessment approaches that recognize and respect the diversity of students' needs, while promoting their engagement and success.

To begin with, it's essential to establish an inclusive learning environment that recognizes and values individual differences. This may involve physical adjustments to the classroom, such as arranging seating to facilitate access for students in wheelchairs, or providing visual aids for hearing-impaired students. Such attention to the learning environment not only promotes student comfort, but also contributes to their sense of belonging and motivation.

One of the key elements of assessment for students with special needs is the personalization of assessment methods. Assessments must be adapted to take account of individual abilities and challenges. However, for students with learning disabilities, it may be beneficial to offer additional testing time, alternative assessment formats or visual and auditory aids. The use of technology, such as assistive writing applications or dictation software, can also support these students in expressing their knowledge and skills [124], [125]

It is also essential to train teachers in inclusive assessment practices. Ongoing training in pupils' specific needs and appropriate assessment methods is crucial to ensure that all teachers feel competent and confident in their ability to assess pupils with diverse needs. Teachers need to be made aware of the different conditions and how to take them into account in their assessment practices. This can include workshops, seminars and online resources that offer concrete strategies for assessing students with special needs.

Another important aspect of inclusive assessment is the involvement of parents and guardians in the process. Parents play a key role in understanding their children's needs and supporting their learning. By involving parents in assessment, teachers can gain valuable insights into students' challenges and successes. Regular meetings, open communication and sharing of learning strategies can strengthen the partnership between school and home, facilitating more consistent support for students.

It is also necessary to assess not only academic performance, but also the socio-emotional well-being of students with special needs. Assessment of socio-emotional skills, such as self-esteem, stress management and resilience, is crucial to the overall development of these students [126]. Appropriate assessment tools, such as questionnaires or individual discussions, can help identify students' emotional needs and put in place appropriate support st$rategies. By recognizing and responding to students' emotional needs, teachers foster a healthy, positive learning environment.

By creating a culture of inclusivity and placing students at the center of the assessment process, teachers help to ensure that every student, whatever their needs, has the opportunity to succeed and flourish in their educational journey.

3.1.2 Strategies for inclusion and equity in evaluation

Strategies for inclusion and equity in assessment are essential to creating an educational environment that respects the diversity of learners and ensures that every student has the opportunity to demonstrate their skills and knowledge. Inclusion and equity are not just limited to access to learning, but also encompass the methods by which students are assessed. Teachers need to adopt varied and adapted approaches to meet the specific needs of each student, while ensuring that assessment criteria are fair and transparent [127], [128].

One of the first strategies for promoting inclusion and equity in assessment is to diversify assessment methods. It's important for teachers to use a range of approaches, including formative, summative, self-, peer and project-based assessments. This gives students many opportunities to show what they've learned, and to express themselves in different ways. For example, some students may excel in written assessments, while others may better demonstrate their understanding through oral presentations or creative projects. By offering a variety of options, teachers create an environment where each student can succeed according to his or her own learning style.

Another key strategy is the implementation of specific accommodations and adaptations for students with special needs. This can include providing extra time for exams [129]modifying the presentation of questions, or using technological tools to aid the expression of ideas: a student with writing difficulties may benefit from the use of dictation software to transcribe his or her answers, while a student with reading difficulties may receive audio versions of the texts to be assessed [130]. These adaptations must be planned in collaboration with educational specialists and parents, to ensure that they meet the specific needs of each student.

It's also essential to promote a culture of inclusivity within the classroom. This means encouraging respect for differences, celebrating diversity and creating an environment where every student feels valued. Teachers can encourage activities to raise awareness of diversity and share personal experiences, enabling students to better understand different perspectives and learn to work together. A positive, inclusive culture not only helps to reduce inequalities, but also fosters collaborative learning that benefits all students.

Inclusive assessment must be a dynamic and adaptable process. Teachers must be ready to adjust their assessment methods in response to student feedback and results. By adopting a reflective approach, teachers can identify gaps in their assessment practices and work to fill them. This implies a willingness to question traditional methods and explore new avenues to ensure that all students have the opportunity to succeed. By integrating these strategies, teachers can create a truly inclusive and equitable assessment system that meets the needs of all students and promotes their success.

3.1.3 Adapting assessment tools

Adapting assessment tools is an essential step in ensuring that all students, whatever their skill level or specific needs, have the opportunity to show what they know and can do. Assessment tools are not just measuring instruments; they play a crucial role in the learning process, providing valuable information to teachers and students alike. Effective assessment must be accessible, fair and relevant, which often requires adjustments and adaptations to meet the diverse needs of learners.

One of the first steps in adapting assessment tools is to assess students' specific needs. This can involve conversations with students, their parents and other professionals, such as education specialists. By understanding each student's strengths and challenges, teachers can better adapt assessment tools so that they are both accessible and appropriate. Integrating technology into assessment tools can play a key role in adapting assessments. Many technological tools offer accessibility features, such as screen readers, dictation software, or applications that make it easier to organize ideas.

Involving students in the process of adapting assessment tools is a valuable approach [24], [131]. Students should be encouraged to share their views on the assessment formats that work best for them, and on the learning strategies that help them succeed. This feedback can guide teachers in modifying their assessment tools and promote greater student autonomy and engagement in their own learning process. Involving students in this process reinforces their sense of responsibility and agentivity in their learning.

Finally, it is essential to regularly evaluate the effectiveness of adapted assessment tools. Teachers should reflect on and analyze how the adaptations they have put in place are actually impacting student performance and engagement. This may involve team discussions, cross-assessments between colleagues, or examining student results to identify the strengths and weaknesses of the assessment tools used. This reflective process enables ongoing adjustments to be made and ensures that assessment tools really do meet students' needs, thus fostering a more inclusive and equitable education system.

3.2 Feedback and communication of results

Feedback and communication of results are essential components of the learning process, playing a crucial role in students' academic and personal development. This chapter discusses the importance of feedback as a tool to help students understand their performance and identify areas for improvement. We begin by exploring why feedback is a fundamental element of learning, highlighting its direct impact on student motivation and progress. Next, we'll look at strategies for giving constructive feedback, which not only informs students about their performance, but also encourages them to adopt a proactive attitude to their learning. Finally, we look at communicating results, emphasizing the importance of conveying this information clearly and constructively to students and their parents. The aim of this chapter is to offer insights and practices that will help teachers to effectively integrate feedback and results communication into their pedagogy, thereby enhancing student engagement and success.

3.2.1 The importance of feedback in the learning process

Feedback plays a central role in the learning process, acting as a lever to improve students' understanding and skills development [132], [133]. It is often defined as information given to a learner about his or her performance, with the aim of guiding learning and encouraging self-improvement. Research has shown that effective feedback can significantly influence learning outcomes, helping students to understand what they have done well and what needs improvement.

One of the key aspects of feedback is that it must be specific, clear and constructive. Students need to know exactly what they have achieved and where they have encountered difficulties. For example, instead of simply saying "good job", a teacher might clarify "your understanding of physics concepts is solid, but it would be useful to review how you apply these concepts in practical situations." This kind of detailed feedback enables students to target their efforts more effectively and adopt learning strategies tailored to their needs [134], [135].

Feedback can also boost student motivation. When they receive positive comments about their efforts and achievements, it can boost their self-confidence and encourage them to continue learning. [136], [137]. Conversely, constructive feedback that highlights areas for improvement, if well formulated, can also be perceived as a learning opportunity rather than a criticism: a teacher might say, "I noticed you had difficulty with that question; let's try together to break down the problem to understand it better." In this way, feedback becomes a tool of encouragement that motivates students to persevere in the face of challenges.

Another essential element of feedback is its frequency and timing. Studies have shown that regular and timely feedback can have a positive impact on learning. When feedback is given soon after a task has been completed, students are better able to make connections between their actions and the results achieved [133]. This enables them to adjust their learning in real time, facilitating a better understanding of the concepts covered [137], [138]. For example, in the context of a group project, frequent feedback on the work accomplished enables students to make modifications and improve their final product before the final assessment.

Feedback should not be a monologue from the teacher; it should also encourage interaction between student and teacher. Encouraging students to ask questions and reflect on feedback promotes a culture of active learning. [139]. Teachers can create opportunities for students to discuss their feedback, enabling them to clarify points that may be unclear and explore strategies for improvement. This interaction not only strengthens students' understanding, but also enables them to become autonomous, reflective learners.

In addition, feedback can also play an important role in the development of transversal skills [140], [141]. By learning to give and receive feedback, students develop essential skills such as communication, collaboration and critical thinking [142]. As an example, in a group work setting, students can learn to provide constructive feedback to their peers, helping them to better understand different perspectives and improve their ability to work as a team. This skill is not only valuable in the school context, but is also essential in professional life [140].

Feedback can also foster a sense of belonging and community within the class. [142]. When students know they are receiving support and constructive feedback from their peers and teachers, it helps to create a positive learning climate. Students are more likely to take risks and express their ideas when they feel safe and supported. This creates an environment where mistakes are seen as a normal and necessary part of the learning process, rather than a failure.

Integrating feedback into the learning process also requires a systematic approach. Teachers need to establish clear expectations for feedback, from both the students' and the teachers' point of view. This can include defining success criteria, creating assessment rubrics and communicating expectations at the outset of a project or assessment. With a shared understanding of objectives and assessment criteria, students are better prepared to receive and integrate feedback into their learning.

Finally, a feedback culture needs to be cultivated within schools. This means that educational leaders must promote positive feedback practices and encourage teachers to adopt assessment strategies that incorporate feedback on a regular and systematic basis [52], [143]. Feedback training and workshops can also be offered to teachers to help them develop effective skills and methods. By embedding feedback into the very fabric of teaching and learning, schools can truly enrich the educational experience and improve learning outcomes for all students.

3.2.2 Strategies for giving constructive feedback

Giving constructive feedback is an essential skill for teachers, as it can transform students' learning experience. For feedback to be truly beneficial, it needs to be both clear and focused, aimed at encouraging reflection and guiding students towards improvement. Several strategies can be implemented to ensure that feedback is constructive and effective.

The first strategy is to use the "sandwich" model to structure the feedback [144], [145], [146]. This model begins with a positive remark, followed by constructive criticism, and ends with another positive note. For example, a teacher might say: "I was really impressed by the way you articulated your ideas in this presentation. However, it would be useful to develop your arguments further with concrete examples. Overall, your ability to communicate clearly is a great asset." This format not only recognizes successes, but also allows criticism to be conveyed in a sensitive manner, reducing the risk of demotivation in the student [145], [147].

Another effective strategy is to make comments based on specific observations rather than general judgments. Instead of saying "it's bad", a teacher should point out precisely what went wrong. For example, "I noticed that you used several technical terms without explaining them, which may have made your presentation difficult for some people to follow." This approach helps the student understand exactly what they need to improve, making feedback more useful and focused [148].

The use of open-ended questions is also a powerful method for stimulating reflection in students. Rather than giving ready-made answers, a teacher can ask questions that prompt students to reflect on their choices and learning processes [149], [150]. For example, by asking "What led you to this conclusion?", the teacher encourages students to analyze their own thinking, which promotes deeper, more autonomous learning [148].

The timing of feedback is another crucial consideration. Providing feedback immediately after a task or assessment allows students to make the connection between their actions and the results [151]. This promotes instant understanding of what needs to be adjusted.

Taking students' emotions into account when delivering feedback is essential[152]. Constructive feedback should not only be about the content, but also about the way it is received. Teachers need to be aware of how their comments can affect student morale. It is therefore also essential to create a climate of trust where students feel comfortable receiving criticism, Teachers can encourage this atmosphere by showing that they see feedback as a learning tool, not a punishment [152]. Explaining to students that feedback is a way of improving their skills and helping them to progress can reduce the anxiety associated with receiving criticism.

In this context, it can also be beneficial to encourage peer-to-peer feedback. When students give each other feedback, it fosters collaborative learning and strengthens their ability to offer constructive criticism. It also helps them learn to receive feedback in a positive way. On the other hand, formulating feedback with a growth perspective can also reinforce its positive impact. By adopting language that emphasizes the potential for improvement and continuous learning, teachers help students adopt a developmental mindset [153]

Finally, it's important to follow up on the feedback given. Teachers need to check whether students have understood the feedback provided, and whether they have incorporated it into their future work. This can be done through one-to-one discussions, questions in subsequent lessons or by examining students' subsequent work. This follow-up shows students that feedback is an ongoing part of their learning process and important to their progress.

3.2.3 Communicating results to students and parents

Communicating results to students and parents is an essential part of the educational process [154], [155]. Not only does it provide an account of academic performance, it also fosters constructive collaboration between school and home. This communication must be clear, transparent and geared towards the continuous improvement of students. Several strategies can be put in place to ensure effective communication of results. The frequency of communication plays a crucial role. Rather than waiting for termly report cards to inform parents of their children's performance, it is beneficial to establish regular points of contact. This can take the form of monthly newsletters, e-mails or individual meetings [156]. These interactions enable teachers to share students' progress, successes and areas for improvement, fostering an open and constructive dialogue. Parents then feel more involved in their child's education and can better support their child's learning at home.

It is also essential to use accessible language when communicating results. Avoiding educational jargon and using simple terms ensures that all parents, whatever their level of education, understand the information provided. For example, instead of saying that a student has achieved a "score of 85 out of 100 in math", it may be more useful to phrase this in terms of goals achieved: "Your child has a good understanding of basic math concepts and is on track to master the skills needed for the next level." This understanding-centred approach facilitates more effective communication and boosts parents' confidence in the education system [157].

The presentation of results must also take into account the emotions of students and parents. When results fall short of expectations, it's crucial to communicate this information with empathy and sensitivity. For example, when announcing a disappointing result, a teacher might address the situation by highlighting the efforts made by the student and suggesting strategies for improving performance in the future. This helps to minimize potential stress and disappointment, encouraging instead an attitude of growth and learning. What's more, by emphasizing effort and progress, even when results are less than ideal, teachers help develop a resilience mentality in students.

Communicating results can also include strategies for engaging students and parents. Involving students in discussing their results is an effective way of helping them become aware of their own learning. For example, teachers can ask students to present their performance at meetings with parents, encouraging them to reflect on their strengths and weaknesses. This approach reinforces personal responsibility and encourages students to take an active part in their education.

In addition, it is important to provide opportunities for one-on-one discussions between teachers and parents. [158], [159]Organizing parent meetings or individual conferences allows parents to ask questions, express concerns and collaborate with teachers to establish action plans tailored to each student. These interactions strengthen the relationship between school and home, establishing an educational partnership that benefits the student. During these meetings, teachers can also offer resources or advice to help parents support their children's learning at home.

Communicating results to students and parents must therefore be a proactive process, centered on dialogue and collaboration. By adopting clear, accessible and empathetic strategies, teachers can not only inform parents of their children's performance, but also encourage them to become actively involved in the educational process. This synergy between school and home is essential to creating a positive and stimulating learning environment, conducive to student success.

Conclusion

Inclusive assessment and constructive feedback are essential pillars for ethical, equitable and sustainable learning. Inclusive assessment recognizes the diversity of abilities and aims to create learning opportunities for every student, especially those with special needs. By adapting assessment tools and methods, teachers ensure that every student has fair conditions conducive to success. Similarly, clear, benevolent feedback enables students to better understand their performance and adjust their learning strategies, thus strengthening their commitment and motivation. Communicating results with both students and parents helps build a collaborative environment, reinforcing everyone's trust and involvement in the educational process.

By integrating inclusive practices and constructive feedback, teachers enrich the learning experience and create a climate where every student is encouraged to progress. This chapter thus calls for continued reflection on the collective responsibility of educators to create accessible, inclusive and stimulating learning environments, emphasizing the importance of benevolent assessment in achieving the educational goals and personal development of each learner.

Chapter 4: Assessment and Digital Innovation

4.1 Student assessment and motivation

Assessment and student motivation are intimately linked, as assessment practices can have a significant impact on students' engagement and attitude towards their learning. This chapter explores this dynamic by first examining the impact of assessment on student motivation, highlighting how different forms of assessment can influence their perceptions, self-confidence and desire to learn. Next, we'll look at specific techniques teachers can use to encourage motivation through assessment, presenting approaches that transform assessment into a positive and motivating tool. Finally, we'll discuss assessment as a personal development tool, highlighting how thoughtful assessment can not only help students acquire knowledge, but also develop personal and social skills essential to their future success. Through this exploration, this chapter aims to provide educators with practical insights and tools for integrating motivation into their assessment practices, thereby fostering more engaged and meaningful learning.

4.1.1 The impact of evaluation on motivation

Assessment plays a central role in students' educational careers, and has a significant impact on their motivation. This influence can be both positive and negative, depending on how assessment is designed, implemented and communicated. Understanding how assessment affects student motivation is crucial to creating a stimulating learning environment conducive to personal and academic development [160].

One of the main factors to consider is the nature of the assessment itself. Formative assessments, which aim to provide feedback on student performance throughout the learning process, tend to encourage intrinsic motivation. These assessments enable students to see their progress, understand their mistakes and engage in a cycle of continuous improvement. For example, when teachers provide constructive feedback and emphasize effort and growth, students are often more motivated to persevere and take on challenges. This creates a positive learning climate where the focus is on learning rather than just getting grades.

On the other hand, summative assessments, which focus on measuring performance at a given point in time, can sometimes generate excessive pressure on students. When perceived as definitive judgments of their ability or worth, they can lead to anxiety, fear of failure and disengagement. For example, students who receive lower grades than expected can develop a performance mentality, where they focus solely on the outcome rather than the learning process. This performance orientation can damage their motivation, leading them to avoid challenges and focus on tasks they feel they can succeed at, rather than exploring learning opportunities.

The way in which assessment results are communicated also plays a crucial role in the impact of assessment on motivation. Communication that focuses on areas for improvement, without acknowledging successes, can demotivate students. It is therefore essential that teachers adopt a balanced approach when presenting results, highlighting both successes and areas for improvement [4], [161]. For example, feedback that highlights progress while offering advice on how to tackle difficulties can encourage students to continue their efforts and feel valued in their learning.

The relationship between teacher and student is also a determining factor in the impact of assessment on motivation. A teacher who establishes a positive connection with his or her students, showing empathy and valuing their efforts, can significantly influence their perception of assessment. Students are more likely to feel motivated and engaged when they believe their teacher cares about their learning and supports them in their challenges. Conversely, a strained or distant relationship can heighten the fear of failure and stress associated with assessments, leading to decreased motivation [162], [163].

Another aspect to consider is how assessments are perceived by the students themselves. Students with a growth mindset, who believe that their abilities can be developed through effort and perseverance, are often more motivated by assessments than those with a fixed mindset, who believe that their intelligence and skills are immutable traits [164], [165]. Thus, teaching students the importance of effort, resilience and learning by doing can have a positive impact on their motivation. Teachers can foster this mindset by celebrating failures as learning opportunities and encouraging students to see challenges as opportunities for growth.

Peer and self-assessment can also have a significant impact on motivation. By actively participating in their own assessment or evaluating their peers, students develop a better understanding of success criteria and strengthen their commitment to their learning. These practices also foster autonomy and responsibility, key elements of intrinsic motivation [69]When students take part in peer assessment, they are not only exposed to different perspectives, but also strengthen their own analytical and critical thinking skills.

Finally, the impact of evaluation on motivation is also influenced by cultural and social context [166], [167]. Parental expectations, educational community norms and school policies can shape the way students perceive assessment [168]. So in environments where academic achievement is highly valued, students may feel extra pressure to perform, which in turn can affect their motivation. It is therefore important for teachers to take these contextual factors into account and adapt their assessment approaches to support all students, creating an inclusive and motivating learning environment [169].

The impact of assessment on motivation is therefore a complex subject that requires in-depth reflection on assessment practices. By adopting learning-centered approaches, fostering positive relationships with students and communicating results constructively, teachers can transform assessment into a powerful tool for encouraging motivation and supporting students' academic and personal development.

4.1.2 Techniques for encouraging motivation through evaluation

Encouraging student motivation through assessment requires the adoption of varied and strategic techniques [4]. These techniques aim to transform assessment into a lever for engagement, self-efficacy and personal satisfaction. By integrating thoughtful assessment methods, teachers can create a learning environment where students feel valued, involved and motivated to achieve their academic goals.

One of the most effective techniques for encouraging motivation is the use of formative assessment. This approach, which involves assessing students throughout the learning process rather than at the end of a module, provides immediate feedback. This feedback helps students identify their strengths and weaknesses, while encouraging them to reflect on their own learning. For example, a teacher might organize regular quizzes or class discussions that allow students to check their understanding of concepts before a summative assessment. By receiving constructive feedback and having the opportunity to improve their skills, students are often more motivated to invest themselves in their learning [4], [160], [170].

Creating a positive and supportive learning environment is essential to motivating students through assessment. Teachers should strive to build a classroom culture where mistakes are seen as learning opportunities rather than failures. Encouraging students to share their difficulties and work together to overcome these challenges can also boost motivation [171]. By setting up study groups or collaborative revision sessions, students can support each other, creating a sense of community and belonging. This positive climate helps build students' confidence and encourages them to take risks in their learning.

Encouraging students to set personal goals and reflect on their progress is essential to maintaining their motivation [172]. Teachers can organize planning sessions where students identify their learning goals and establish concrete steps to achieve them. Students can thus be invited to reflect on the skills they wish to develop and draw up an action plan to achieve them. This practice not only fosters personal responsibility, but also helps students see their progress over time, reinforcing their motivation to keep up their efforts.

Techniques for encouraging motivation through assessment are varied and can be adapted to suit the specific needs of students and the learning context. By incorporating formative assessments, setting clear objectives, creating a positive environment, encouraging self-assessment, using peer assessment, offering choices and encouraging reflection on progress, teachers can transform the assessment process into a powerful motivator. In so doing, they help to develop learners who are autonomous, committed and ready to meet the challenges of their educational journey.

4.1.3 Evaluation as a tool for personal development

Assessment, often seen simply as a means of measuring academic performance, has considerable potential as a tool for personal development. Indeed, when thoughtfully designed and implemented, assessment can play a crucial role in students' individual growth, helping them to better understand their abilities, build self-confidence and develop essential life skills [173], [174].

Firstly, assessment can promote self-awareness. By taking part in formative and summative assessments, students are encouraged to reflect on their knowledge and skills. This reflection enables them to identify their strengths and weaknesses. When students receive feedback on an assignment, they may realize that they excel in certain areas, such as writing, while needing improvement in others, such as critical analysis. This awareness is an essential step in personal development, as it encourages students to take a proactive approach to their learning. In this way, they learn to set realistic goals and work on their areas for improvement, fostering a sense of autonomy and commitment [4].

In addition, assessment can serve as a springboard for the development of resilience [175]. Faced with evaluative challenges, students must learn to manage stress and pressure, persevere in the face of failure and develop a growth mindset. A student who scores below expectations may be prompted to reflect on the reasons for this result and develop an action plan for improvement [176]. This process of learning through failure is essential, as it teaches students that mistakes are not ends in themselves, but opportunities to learn and grow. By cultivating this resilience, students prepare themselves not only to overcome academic challenges, but also those of everyday life.

Assessment can also encourage the development of interpersonal and teamwork skills. Group assessment activities, such as collaborative projects or presentations, offer students the opportunity to work together, share ideas and learn to manage conflict. Through these interactions, students develop essential skills such as communication, negotiation and leadership [177]. A group project in which each member is required to contribute to part of the presentation not only reinforces academic knowledge, but also cultivates positive relationships between students. This social dimension of assessment helps prepare students for a collaborative working environment in the future.

Assessment as a tool for personal development also manifests itself in the encouragement of self-regulation. When students are involved in the assessment process, through self-assessment or peer assessment, they develop critical skills that enable them to manage their own learning [178], [179]. By being responsible for their own assessment, students learn to establish criteria for success, reflect on their performance and adjust their learning strategies accordingly. This ability to self-regulate is not only beneficial for their academic career, but is also crucial for their long-term personal and professional development.

Assessment can also be used to boost students' intrinsic motivation, enabling them to set meaningful, personal learning goals [180]. By offering choices in the assessment process, such as the format of presentation or the topic of a project, students feel more invested and motivated: a student who is passionate about a particular topic will be more motivated to investigate further and invest themselves in their work [161]. This autonomy of choice also strengthens their commitment to their learning, which is a key factor in their personal development.

Another important aspect is how assessment can contribute to the development of a lifelong learning mentality. By instilling a positive assessment culture that values effort and improvement over performance alone, teachers can encourage students to embrace the concept of lifelong learning. By celebrating progress and emphasizing the importance of effort, students are encouraged to view their educational journey as an ongoing process. This not only fosters their personal development, but also prepares them for a professional career in which learning and adaptation are essential [181].

Assessment, when used strategically and thoughtfully, becomes a powerful personal development tool for students. It fosters self-awareness, builds resilience, improves interpersonal skills, encourages self-regulation and enhances intrinsic motivation. By integrating these dimensions into the assessment process, teachers can help students develop not only as learners, but also as individuals, prepared to face life's challenges with confidence and determination.

4.2 Evaluation in a digital context

Assessment in a digital context represents a major evolution in contemporary educational practices, offering new possibilities for measuring student learning in a more interactive and adaptive way. This chapter examines the various digital tools available for assessment, which facilitate not only the creation of more diverse and engaging assessments, but also the collection and analysis of student performance. We'll also look at the benefits and challenges of online assessment, exploring how this modality can enrich the learning experience while raising crucial questions about the fairness, security and integrity of assessments. Finally, we will look at the use of data from digital assessments to improve pedagogical practices, highlighting the importance of a data-driven approach to adjusting teaching and assessment strategies. This chapter aims to provide educators with practical insights and reflections on how digital assessment can be effectively integrated into their daily practice.

4.2.1 Digital assessment tools

The integration of digital tools into the assessment process has transformed traditional methods, offering new opportunities to measure students' skills and knowledge in a more dynamic and engaging way [34], [182], [183]. Digital tools not only facilitate assessment, but also enrich the learning experience. In this context, a variety of tools and technologies are emerging, each with distinct features that can meet the varied needs of teachers and students.

Online evaluation platforms are among the most widely used tools [183]. They enable teachers to create, distribute and grade tests quickly and efficiently. Platforms such as Google Forms, Quizizz and Kahoot! offer interactive features that engage students while facilitating the assessment process. [184]. For example, Kahoot! uses interactive quizzes where students can participate in real time, fostering a competitive and stimulating environment. These tools also enable rapid analysis of results, providing teachers with valuable statistics on student performance, enabling them to adapt their teaching accordingly.

Another important aspect of digital tools for assessment is the possibility of using electronic portfolios [185]. These platforms enable students to collect and organize their work, projects and reflections throughout their academic career. Tools such as Seesaw and Mahara enable students to document their learning and present their achievements in a way that goes beyond simple grades. E-portfolios also encourage self-assessment and reflection, as students can look back on previous work and assess their progress over time. This approach encourages a more holistic view of assessment, where students are actively involved in their learning process [185], [186], [187], [188].

Peer review tools also represent a significant innovation in the digital field [189], [190]. Platforms such as Peergrade or Turnitin enable students to assess the work of their peers, which not only fosters collaborative learning, but also a deeper understanding of assessment criteria [191]. This type of assessment encourages students to develop critical and analytical skills, while strengthening their ability to give and receive constructive feedback. In addition, peer assessment helps to create a more participative and inclusive classroom climate, where students feel valued and responsible for their collective learning.

Adaptive assessments are another key development in the digital field. These systems use algorithms to adjust the difficulty of questions based on student responses, allowing for personalized and targeted assessment [192], [193]. Tools such as Knewton and DreamBox Learning adapt to each student's skill level, offering assessments that are not only accurate but also motivating. This type of dynamic assessment allows teachers to gain an overview of students' skills, while offering students challenges that match their level of understanding [194].

Finally, data analysis tools play a crucial role in digital assessment. The use of analytics software enables teachers to track student performance, identify trends and make informed decisions about instruction [195]. Tools such as Tableau or Power BI allow assessment data to be visualized, making it easier to understand student results and progress. These analyses can be used to adapt teaching strategies, addressing specific student needs and continuously improving the educational process [196].

Digital assessment tools offer unprecedented opportunities to enrich the learning experience. By integrating online assessment platforms, e-portfolios, peer reviews, serious games, adaptive assessments and data analysis tools, teachers can create an interactive and engaging learning environment [197]. This digital transformation goes beyond simply measuring academic performance; it also fosters active, collaborative learning, prepares students for an ever-changing digital world and enables them to develop essential skills for their future.

4.2.2 Online evaluation: benefits and challenges

Online assessment has become an essential component of the modern educational landscape, offering both significant benefits and considerable challenges. This mode of assessment, which uses digital platforms to administer and mark tests and assessments, has developed widely, not least in response to the need for adaptability in the face of situations such as the COVID-19 pandemic. The benefits of online assessment are varied, and affect both teachers and students.

One of the main advantages of online assessment is the flexibility it offers. Students can take tests at their convenience, enabling better time management, especially for those with commitments outside school [198], [199]. This flexibility is also beneficial for teachers, who can design assessments that can be administered at different times, depending on students' needs. What's more, online assessment tools enable testing to be carried out remotely, thus widening access to education for students who, for geographical or personal reasons, cannot be physically present in a classroom.

Another major advantage is the speed of correction and feedback. Online assessment platforms often offer automated features that enable multiple-choice tests to be marked in real time, and results to be provided instantly to students. This significantly reduces the time teachers spend on marking, enabling them to concentrate more on teaching and supporting students. This speed of feedback is crucial to the learning process, as it enables students to immediately understand their errors and adapt their learning strategies accordingly [200], [201], [202], [203].

Online assessment also offers diversified and innovative assessment possibilities. Teachers can create multimedia tests incorporating videos, images and interactive simulations, making assessment more engaging and relevant. For example, a science test could include a video of an experiment to be analyzed, which would not be possible in a traditional paper format. This diversity enriches the assessment experience and allows students to demonstrate their skills in a more authentic way.

However, despite these advantages, online evaluation also presents several challenges [204]. One of the biggest is that of equity and access. Not all students have equal access to digital technologies and the Internet, which can create inequalities in the assessment process [205]. Students from disadvantaged backgrounds may find themselves at a disadvantage if they do not have access to a computer or a stable Internet connection [206]. This raises questions about the fairness of student outcomes in an online assessment environment, and highlights the need for alternative solutions to ensure equitable access.

The security and integrity of online assessments is another major challenge. The risks of fraud and cheating are amplified in a digital environment, where students may be tempted to use unauthorized resources during a test. Teachers must therefore be vigilant and implement security measures, such as using remote monitoring systems or designing assessments that minimize the possibility of cheating [206], [207], [208]. In addition, the management of students' personal data must be a priority, in order to guarantee the protection of their privacy and comply with data protection regulations.

Another challenge concerns the quality of assessments. Although digital tools enable the creation of a variety of tests, it is essential that these assessments are well designed and aligned with learning objectives. Teachers must ensure that online assessments actually measure the skills and knowledge they are designed to assess. This requires adequate training for teachers in the use of digital tools and the design of effective assessments. Without this, there is a high risk of generating unreliable or irrelevant assessments [34], [206], [209].

Finally, adapting to the digital format can be a challenge for some students. While many students become familiar with digital technologies, others may have difficulty navigating online environments. This difficulty can lead to additional stress or anxiety during assessments, affecting their performance. Teachers need to be aware of these variabilities and offer adequate support to help all students feel comfortable and confident with online assessment [210].

Online assessment offers undeniable advantages in terms of flexibility, speed and innovation. However, it also brings with it challenges relating to fairness, security, assessment quality and student adaptation. To take full advantage of online assessment, it's crucial that teachers and educational establishments address these challenges proactively, putting strategies in place to ensure that all students benefit from fair and meaningful assessment in a digital environment.

4.2.3 Using data to improve evaluation

The use of data in assessment has become an essential practice for improving educational processes and optimizing student learning [211]. Data collected from digital assessments provide valuable information on student performance, learning behaviors, as well as the effectiveness of implemented pedagogical strategies [5], [211]. By analyzing this data, teachers can identify trends, adapt their teaching and, ultimately, support students in a more targeted way.

A fundamental aspect of using data is the ability to measure student progress on an ongoing basis. Online assessments enable data to be collected at every stage of learning, whether through quizzes, exams or projects. These assessments make it possible to track not only overall results, but also the specific skills that each student has mastered or still needs to develop. For example, if a student shows difficulties in a particular area, teachers can intervene quickly to provide targeted support, whether through remediation, tutoring or additional resources [211], [212].

Assessment data can also be used to identify gaps and strengths in the curriculum. By analyzing test results at an aggregate level, educators can spot trends that highlight areas where students are experiencing general difficulties [212]. This can lead to a revision of course content or teaching methods, to better meet students' needs. For example, if results show that the majority of students fail questions relating to a fundamental concept, this may indicate that the concept has not been taught in a sufficiently clear or engaging way.

In addition, the use of data can help personalize learning [213]. With the information gathered, teachers can better understand each student's preferences and learning styles. As a result, they can design assessments and teaching activities to meet individual student needs. For example, if a student excels at visual learning, the teacher can integrate visual elements into assessments to make content more accessible and engaging. This individualized approach not only promotes student engagement, but also contributes to a significant improvement in student performance.

The analysis of educational data is not limited to the evaluation of student performance; it also includes reflection on teaching practices. Teachers can use analysis tools to examine the effectiveness of their own teaching strategies. By comparing student results before and after the implementation of a new teaching method, they can determine whether it has a positive impact on learning. For example, if a teacher introduces a project-based learning method and sees a significant improvement in student performance on subsequent assessments, this may confirm the effectiveness of this approach [214], [215], [216].

Another important aspect of using data to improve assessment is the implementation of data-driven feedback systems [217]. Teachers can take advantage of assessment results to give more specific and relevant feedback to students. Rather than providing general feedback, teachers can refer to specific data to discuss student progress, recurring errors and areas for work. This feedback approach, rooted in concrete data, helps students understand exactly where they are in their learning and what they need to do to improve.

Data can also play a crucial role in the development of student support programs [218], [219]. By identifying students with difficulties on the basis of assessment data, schools can implement targeted interventions, such as tutoring programs, support groups or specific workshops. For example, if the data show that a group of students is struggling in math, the school can organize remediation sessions to specifically address problematic concepts. This enables a proactive approach to education, where problems are identified and addressed before they become major obstacles to learning.

It is also essential to stress that the use of data in evaluation requires adequate training for teachers. To get the most out of analysis tools and data collection platforms, educators need to be trained not only on how to use these tools, but also on how to interpret and act on the data. A thorough understanding of data enables them to make informed choices that will positively influence student learning. Ongoing training and resources must be made available to support teachers in this process.

Finally, the ethical use of data in assessment must be a priority. Protecting students' privacy and using data responsibly are major concerns in the digital context. Schools need to put in place clear policies on data collection, storage and use to ensure the security of student information. This not only contributes to the confidence of students and parents, but also to the creation of a positive and safe learning environment.

Integrating data into the assessment process opens up numerous possibilities for improving learning and teaching. By using data to track student progress, adapt teaching methods, personalize learning and provide constructive feedback, teachers can not only improve assessment but also enrich the overall educational experience. What's more, with the right training and an ethical approach, the use of data can transform the educational landscape, making assessment more effective and meaningful for all involved.

4.3 Reflections on the future of evaluation

The landscape of educational assessment is constantly evolving, influenced by technological, socio-cultural and pedagogical factors that are redefining learning and assessment expectations. This chapter looks at reflections on the future of assessment, beginning by exploring the current trends shaping the practice. We'll look at how approaches such as formative assessment, the use of digital technologies and learner-centered methods are emerging as effective solutions to meet the varied needs of students. We will then discuss the challenges and opportunities of assessment in a changing world, considering the implications of rapid changes in society, the job market and educational expectations. Finally, we will propose practical perspectives and recommendations for teachers, to help them navigate this changing dynamic and adapt their assessment practices accordingly. This chapter aims to inspire proactive thinking about the future of assessment, and to encourage educators to prepare for tomorrow's challenges while maximizing learning opportunities for their students.

4.3.1 Current valuation trends

Current trends in educational assessment reflect a move towards more learner-centered practices, incorporating innovative approaches and taking into account the diverse needs of students. These trends are shaped by factors such as technological advances, pedagogical research and the demands of an ever-changing world. Against this backdrop, a number of trends are emerging that are redefining the way assessment is conceived and implemented [2], [35], [220].

One of the major trends is the emphasis on formative assessment [50], [221]. Unlike summative assessment, which focuses on the final judgment of students' achievements, formative assessment aims to provide continuous feedback throughout the learning process. This approach enables students to understand their strengths and weaknesses in real time, fostering autonomous, proactive learning. Teachers use a variety of tools and techniques, such as online quizzes, class discussions and self-assessments, to gather data on student progress and adjust their teaching accordingly. This trend towards formative assessment transforms the teacher's role into that of facilitator, able to accompany each student on his or her learning journey.

Another significant trend is the integration of peer and self-assessment. These methods encourage students to actively engage in their own learning process by evaluating their own work and that of their peers [222]. Peer assessment develops critical and analytical skills, while strengthening collaboration and dialogue between students. Self-assessment, on the other hand, enables students to become aware of their own learning, set goals and evaluate their progress in relation to these goals. These practices foster students' autonomy and give them the tools they need to become reflective and responsible learners [223].

The increased use of technology in the assessment process is also a significant trend. [182]. Digital tools not only facilitate data collection and analysis, but also enable more engaging and interactive assessments. Online assessment platforms offer features such as adaptive quizzes, which adjust the difficulty of questions according to students' responses, and immersive simulations, which enable skills to be practiced in realistic environments. The accessibility of these tools promotes flexible learning, where students can work at their own pace, and this opens up new avenues for authentic assessment [224].

The personalization of assessment is another trend that is gaining in importance. Thanks to technological advances and data analysis, teachers are now able to design assessments that take into account the individual needs of each student. By adapting assessment modalities to students' learning styles, interests and skill levels, teachers can ensure a more inclusive and effective learning experience. This personalized approach not only increases students' motivation, but also improves their engagement and performance [225].

At the same time, there is a growing emphasis on cross-disciplinary skills in assessment processes. Skills such as collaboration, communication, critical thinking and creativity are increasingly recognized as essential elements to be assessed in modern education [226]. Educational establishments are striving to integrate these skills into their assessments, setting up interdisciplinary projects and practical activities that enable students to demonstrate their ability to apply their knowledge in real-life contexts. This reflects a holistic vision of education, which goes beyond the mere acquisition of theoretical knowledge.

Inclusive assessment, aimed at meeting the needs of students with special needs, is also a growing trend. Educators are becoming aware of the importance of adapting assessment practices to ensure that all students, whatever their challenges or abilities, can participate fully in the learning process. This may involve using adapted materials, modifying assessment criteria or offering different ways of expressing knowledge. This approach fosters a learning environment that is equitable and respectful of diversity [227], [228].

Finally, thinking about the purpose of assessment is evolving. Increasingly, assessment is seen as a tool for personal development, rather than simply a means of sanctioning errors or grading students. Educators and students alike recognize that assessment must be used to enrich the learning process and promote a culture of success and growth. This includes the implementation of constructive feedback practices, where the focus is on progress made and steps ahead rather than past mistakes.

4.3.2 Assessment in a changing world

Assessment in a changing world is an exciting challenge that requires constant adaptation to new social, economic and technological realities. In a context where the knowledge and skills required by the job market are changing rapidly, education systems need to re-evaluate and redefine their assessment methods to meet these new demands. This means revising learning objectives, assessment methods and success criteria, while taking into account the diverse needs of students.

One of the defining features of this changing world is the acceleration of digital transformation [229]. Digital technologies, including artificial intelligence, e-learning and data analysis tools, are radically changing the way assessment is designed and implemented. For example, online assessment platforms enable tests to be tailored to students' individual abilities, providing a more personalized and effective experience. This technology also enables instant feedback, which is essential for the ongoing development of skills. In a digital environment, students can receive immediate feedback on their performance, enabling them to better understand their mistakes and adjust their learning accordingly[230].

In this context, assessment must evolve to value not only theoretical knowledge, but also practical and cross-disciplinary skills. The ability to solve problems, work in teams and adapt to changing environments is increasingly recognized as essential for success in the professional world. Assessment systems therefore need to incorporate methods that measure these skills, such as collaborative projects, case studies and simulations. These assessment methods encourage an authentic approach, where students are confronted with real-life situations that prepare them for the challenges of the future.

In addition, evaluation must also take into account cultural diversity and social inequalities. [231]. As societies become increasingly multicultural, it is crucial that evaluation systems are inclusive and equitable. This means that they must strive to reduce bias and adapt assessment criteria to meet the needs of all students, whatever their socio-economic or cultural background. Educators must be trained to design assessments that take this diversity into account, using flexible approaches that respect individual differences [232].

In addition, the impact of climate change and environmental issues on education and assessment is also an aspect to consider. Skills related to sustainability, critical thinking about environmental challenges and social responsibility need to be integrated into learning objectives. Assessment systems must then be able to evaluate these skills, encouraging students to reflect on their role as global citizens. Projects dealing with environmental issues, research into sustainable solutions or community action can serve as solid foundations for such assessments [233], [234].

At the same time, remote assessment has gained considerable momentum, not least because of recent global events such as the COVID-19 pandemic [235]. This shift has revealed inequalities in access to education and highlighted the need for assessment systems that work effectively, whatever the mode of delivery. Institutions must now consider hybrid solutions that combine face-to-face and distance learning, while ensuring that assessments are fair and reliable in all contexts [236].

Assessment in a changing world must also take into account the expectations of stakeholders, including employers and parents. Employers are increasingly looking for graduates with practical and adaptive skills, able to work in diverse and changing environments [237]. Consequently, education systems need to connect with industries and integrate their expectations into assessment programs. This can include partnering with companies to develop assessments that reflect the skills in demand on the job market.

the issue of ethical responsibility and transparency in assessment becomes crucial. As assessment technologies evolve, it is essential to ensure that student data is protected and used ethically. Educators, institutions and decision-makers must commit to high standards of confidentiality and data security, while ensuring that assessment systems are accessible and fair to all.

4.3.3 Prospects and recommendations for teachers

Assessment perspectives and recommendations for teachers need to be addressed in the context of a reflection on the evolution of education and the skills required by students in a rapidly changing world [238]. To achieve this, it is crucial that teachers adopt a proactive approach, incorporating assessment methods that are both relevant and adaptable. This starts with an awareness of the different issues facing assessment today, including technological developments, societal expectations, and the diverse needs of learners.

Firstly, teachers need to engage in ongoing training to keep abreast of the latest research in evaluation and pedagogy. [239]. This training can take various forms, such as workshops, seminars, or even communities of practice within schools [240]. By immersing themselves in new trends and methods, teachers will be better prepared to integrate a variety of assessment approaches, ranging from formative assessment to peer and self-assessment. This will help them not only to better assess students' skills, but also to promote a positive and dynamic learning climate [20].

Secondly, teachers should adopt a learner-centred approach in their assessment practices. This means taking into account the needs, interests and learning styles of each individual student. By personalizing assessment methods, such as offering different modalities (written, oral, practical) and integrating collaborative projects, teachers can create more inclusive and engaging learning experiences. This personalization also fosters student motivation and engagement, by actively involving them in their own learning process [241], [242].

Third, it is essential that teachers use digital tools and educational technologies to enrich their assessment practices [131], [243].

Integrating these tools can open up new possibilities for collecting data, analyzing performance and providing rapid feedback. Teachers can take advantage of online assessment platforms to create adaptive assessments that respond to students' individual abilities [244]. By using learning data to refine their teaching methods, teachers can better meet their students' needs and improve the effectiveness of their assessment.

In addition, it is important for teachers to develop clear and transparent success criteria [99], [245]. These criteria should be shared with students at the start of a module or project, to inform them of the expectations and goals to be achieved. By making these criteria visible and accessible, teachers help students to better understand what is expected of them, and this also enables them to set personal goals. In addition, well-defined grading scales can help ensure fair and objective assessment, reducing subjective bias.

Another crucial recommendation for teachers is to encourage constructive and continuous feedback [246]. Feedback should not be seen solely as a final assessment, but as a central part of the learning process. By providing regular, detailed feedback, teachers can guide students in their learning efforts and help them identify their strengths and areas for improvement. This helps to create a culture of positive feedback where students feel supported on their journey.

Teachers should also consider collaborating with other education professionals to enrich their assessment practices [247], [248]. By sharing resources, ideas and experiences, they can develop more comprehensive and effective approaches to assessment. Exchanges with colleagues, whether within the same school or through wider networks, provide a diversity of perspectives that can fuel innovation in assessment.

Finally, it is imperative that teachers take account of issues of inclusion and equity in their assessment practices [249]. This means adapting tools and methods to meet the needs of all students, especially those with special needs. Teachers need to be trained in inclusive assessment practices and the use of adaptations that ensure every student can participate fully and have a fair chance to succeed. By creating a respectful and equitable learning environment, teachers contribute to building a more inclusive society.

Overall, the perspectives and recommendations for teachers on assessment emphasize the importance of a reflective and adaptive approach. By integrating learner-centered practices, using digital tools, clarifying success criteria and promoting constructive feedback, teachers can transform their assessment methods to better meet the challenges of today's world. It is by adopting these principles that teachers will be able to prepare students to successfully navigate an ever-changing future.

Conclusion

Assessment, whether motivational, digital or future-oriented, plays a crucial role in creating a dynamic learning environment that is adapted to students' needs. The impact of assessment on motivation underlines the importance of a caring approach, which goes beyond the simple measurement of performance to support students' personal development and engagement in their learning. Digital tools enrich this process by making assessments more accessible and diversified, enabling more personalized learning that responds to individual styles and needs. However, these innovations require thoughtful use to ensure fair and reliable results.

In the face of societal and technological change, it is becoming essential for educators to adopt flexible, innovative assessment practices that encourage a proactive, integrative vision of assessment. This chapter invites teachers to consider assessment not just as a measurement tool, but as a lever for growth, offering students opportunities to thrive in a constantly changing world. By adopting these perspectives, educators can not only improve the effectiveness of their assessments, but also prepare students to become autonomous learners and engaged citizens, capable of meeting tomorrow's challenges.

General conclusion

This book offers a comprehensive exploration of assessment in the contemporary educational context, highlighting its essential role as a driver of learning and student success. Through its various chapters, we have addressed the multiple dimensions of assessment, from definitions and objectives to digital tools and inclusive practices, feedback techniques and the importance of motivation. Each section has sought to emphasize not only the need for rigorous, objective assessment, but also the importance of a humane, learner-centered approach.

One of the key conclusions of this book is that assessment should not be seen simply as a measuring tool, but rather as a dynamic, interactive process that promotes active learning. By integrating practices such as formative assessment, peer assessment and self-assessment, we have seen how students can become active participants in their own learning, developing a better understanding of their strengths and weaknesses. This fosters a culture of continuous learning, where mistakes are seen as an opportunity for improvement rather than a failure.

In addition, the importance of inclusivity and equity in assessment practices was highlighted as a moral and educational imperative. In an increasingly diverse school environment, it is crucial that assessment tools are adapted to meet the varied needs of students, ensuring that everyone has an equal opportunity to succeed. By promoting practices that value diversity and take into account students' specificities, we contribute to creating fairer and more accessible learning environments.

The book also highlighted the role of new technologies in the evolution of assessment. The use of digital tools offers unprecedented opportunities to diversify assessment methods, make the process more engaging and provide valuable data to guide pedagogical decisions. However, it is essential to approach these innovations with discernment, ensuring that they serve to enrich the educational experience rather than replace it. We also looked at current trends and future prospects for assessment, underlining the importance of remaining adaptable in the face of rapid changes in the world of education. Teachers, trainers and decision-makers need to continually reflect on their assessment practices to ensure that they remain relevant and effective in an ever-changing context. The recommendations made throughout this book are designed to encourage critical reflection and inspire concrete action to improve evaluation practices.

Overall, this book aspires to be a valuable resource for all those involved in education. By fostering a thoughtful, inclusive and learner-centered approach, we can transform assessment into a powerful lever for student learning and success. Whether in the classroom, in a digital environment or through collaborative practices, every player in education has a role to play in creating an assessment system that values the potential of every student and prepares future generations to meet the challenges of an ever-changing world.

References

[1] Laila Laila, Alawiyah Nabila, and Eka Widyanti, "Konsep Dasar Evaluasi Pembelajaran," *jmpai*, vol. 2, no. 5, pp. 252-262, Jul. 2024, doi: 10.61132/jmpai.v2i5.536.

[2] R. Meylani, "A Comparative Analysis of Traditional and Modern Approaches to Assessment and Evaluation in Education," *Batı Anadolu Eğitim Bilimleri Dergisi*, vol. 15, no. 1, pp. 520-555, Apr. 2024, doi: 10.51460/baebd.1386737.

[3] M. Zhou, "Significance of Assessment in Learning: The Role of Educational Assessment Tools," *Sci Insights Educ Front*, vol. 18, no. 2, pp. 2881-2883, Oct. 2023, doi: 10.15354/sief.23.co215.

[4] I. Magdalena, M. G. Andreani, S. Nurhasanah, and Z. M. Ushaybiah, "DAMPAK PENILAIAN UNTUK PEMBELAJARAN TERHADAP MOTIVASI DAN KETERLIBATAN SISWA," *JRPP*, vol. 2, no. 1, pp. 104-111, Jun. 2023, doi: 10.55047/jrpp.v2i1.450.

[5] H. H. Sievertsen, "Assessments in Education," in *Oxford Research Encyclopedia of Economics and Finance*, Oxford University Press, 2023. doi: 10.1093/acrefore/9780190625979.013.846.

[6] A. G. B. Md Din, M. A. R. Bin Zabidin, A. R. Moawad Ali Tahawi, O. B. Md Din, and F. Aawi, "Educational Assessment: Its Types and Outcomes: A Bibliometric Analytical Study," *IJARBSS*, vol. 13, no. 11, p. Pages 1599-1618, Nov. 2023, doi: 10.6007/IJARBSS/v13-i11/19516.

[7] A. Y. M. Oñate, J. S. C. Molina, L. C. N. Borja, D. J. D. Ojeda, and J. J. D. Carpio, "Theoretical Conceptions about Formative Assessment as a Teaching Tool to Transform Educational Quality," *Intl. J. Rel.* vol. 5, no. 11, pp. 3534-3542, Jul. 2024, doi: 10.61707/ddn9fc82.

[8] S. S. F. J. Jannah and Eka Widyanti, "Assessment of Knowledge Competency Achievement," *JSRET*, vol. 3, no. 2, pp. 881-889, Jun. 2024, doi: 10.58526/jsret.v3i2.429.

[9] E. Gološ, "Measuring instruments and quality of student achievements," *PS*, vol. 12, no. 13, pp. 111-121, Sep. 2023, doi: 10.52580/issn.2232-8556.2023.12.13.111.

[10] P. Black and D. Wiliam, "Inside the Black Box: Raising Standards through Classroom Assessment," *Phi Delta Kappan*, vol. 92, no. 1, pp. 81-90, Sep. 2010, doi: 10.1177/003172171009200119.

[11] M. Heritage, "Formative Assessment: What Do Teachers Need to Know and Do?," *Phi Delta Kappan*, vol. 89, no. 2, pp. 140-145, Oct. 2007, doi: 10.1177/003172170708900210.

[12] J. Hattie and H. Timperley, "The Power of Feedback," *Review of Educational Research*, vol. 77, no. 1, pp. 81-112, Mar. 2007, doi: 10.3102/003465430298487.

[13] M. Newmann Valgueiro, I. Semeão Prazeres, and D. De Oliveira Quaresma, "CONTRIBUTIONS OF INSTITUTIONAL ASSESSMENT FOR THE PLANNING AND MANAGEMENT OF OTHER KNOWLEDGE," *GEI*, vol. 5, no. 01, pp. 107-129, Jan. 2024, doi: 10.51249/gei.v5i01.1849.

[14] *Making Sense of Data-Driven Decision Making in Education: Evidence from Recent RAND Research*. RAND Corporation, 2006. doi: 10.7249/OP170.

[15] Copper Frances Giloth and J. Tanant, "User Experiences in Three Approaches to a Visit to a 3D Labyrinthe of Versailles," 2015, *Unpublished*. doi: 10.13140/RG.2.1.4739.4406.

[16] B. J. Zimmerman, "Becoming a Self-Regulated Learner: An Overview," *Theory Into Practice*, vol. 41, no. 2, pp. 64-70, May 2002, doi: 10.1207/s15430421tip4102_2.

[17] H. Andrade and Y. Du, "Student responses to criteria-referenced self-assessment," *Assessment & Evaluation in Higher Education*, vol. 32, no. 2, pp. 159-181, Apr. 2007, doi: 10.1080/02602930600801928.

[18] E. Panadero and J. Alonso-Tapia, "¿Cómo autorregulan nuestros alumnos? Modelo de Zimmerman sobre estrategias de aprendizaje," *analesps*, vol. 30, no. 2, pp. 450-462, May 2014, doi: 10.6018/analesps.30.2.167221.

[19] D. H. Schunk and J. A. Greene, Eds, *Handbook of Self-Regulation of Learning and Performance*, 2nd ed. Routledge, 2017. doi: 10.4324/9781315697048.

[20] F. Gratani, L. M. Capolla, L. Giannandrea, and P. G. Rossi, "Rethinking assessment practices in schools. A research-training

pathway to foster assessment as learning," *EDUCATION SCIENCES AND SOCIETY*, no. 1, pp. 81-99, Jul. 2023, doi: 10.3280/ess1-2023oa16050.

[21] R. Tammaro and D. Gragnaniello, "Sustainable Assessment as a device to prepare learners for the future," *Form@re*, vol. 24, no. 1, pp. 271-279, Mar. 2024, doi: 10.36253/form-15624.

[22] E. C. Wylie, "Assessment Research and Practices to Advance Human Learning," in *International Handbook on Education Development in Asia-Pacific*, W. O. Lee, P. Brown, A. L. Goodwin, and A. Green, Eds., Singapore: Springer Nature Singapore, 2023, pp. 1-20. doi: 10.1007/978-981-16-2327-1_117-1.

[23] N. J. Rao and S. Banerjee, "Classroom Assessment in Higher Education," *Higher Education for the Future*, vol. 10, no. 1, pp. 11-30, Jan. 2023, doi: 10.1177/23476311221143231.

[24] W. A. Tarihoran and D. K. Nasution, "A Probe into the Impact of Teachers Assessment on Students Engagement in EFL Learning: Views From EFL School Teachers," *jetl*, vol. 6, no. 2, pp. 23-38, Jun. 2024, doi: 10.51178/jetl.v6i2.1841.

[25] F. Arifin, "The Relationship between Diagnostic Assessment and Student Motivation Aspects in the Merdeka curriculum," *armada*, vol. 2, no. 1, pp. 12-20, Mar. 2024, doi: 10.59613/armada.v2i1.2856.

[26] Badrun Kholid, Arif Rahman, and Lalu Ari Irawan, "Implementing Diagnostic Assessment in Designing Differentiated Learning for English Language Learning at the Junior High Schools," *JOLLS. Lang. Liter. Studies*, vol. 4, no. 2, pp. 445-458, Jun. 2024, doi: 10.36312/jolls.v4i2.1934.

[27] S. Kumar, "Impact of Assessment on Childhood Education Theories and Practice:," in *Advances in Early Childhood and K-12 Education*, M. Badea and M. Suditu, Eds., IGI Global, 2024, pp. 84-101. doi: 10.4018/979-8-3693-0956-8.ch004.

[28] G. S. Maxwell, "Assessment and accountability global trends and future directions in 21st century competencies," in *International Encyclopedia of Education(Fourth Edition)*, Elsevier, 2023, pp. 313-323. doi: 10.1016/B978-0-12-818630-5.09069-2.

[29] Nurmaliati, Atika Ulya Akmali, and Azmi Asra, "Using Assessment As Learning With Active Feedback: Effect On Student Achievement," *IJEET*, vol. 2, no. 2, pp. 246-256, Apr. 2024, doi: 10.61991/ijeet.v2i2.46.

[30] C. A. Dwyer, Ed, *The Future of Assessment: Shaping Teaching and Learning*, 1st ed. Routledge, 2017. doi: 10.4324/9781315086545.

[31] Korean Society for Holistic Convergence Education, W. S. Choi, and H. Kil, "An Analysis on the Need of Teacher-Parent for Student Evaluation Information," *Korean Soc Holist Converg Edu*, vol. 27, no. 3, pp. 1-19, Sep. 2023, doi: 10.35184/kshce.2023.27.3.1.

[32] I. Morawska, "Ocenianie w szkole jako komunikacja interakcyjna," *en*, no. 4, p. 195, Dec. 2019, doi: 10.17951/en.2019.4.195-211.

[33] T. V. Zykova, A. A. Kytmanov, E. A. Khalturin, Yu. V. Vaynshteyn, and M. V. Noskov, "The algorithm for analysis and evaluation of educational programs curricula," *Informatika i obrazovanie*, vol. 39, no. 1, pp. 52-64, Apr. 2024, doi: 10.32517/0234-0453-2024-39-1-52-64.

[34] L. Sembiring and S. S. Sembiring, "Practical Application of Assessment Theories for English Teacher through Digital Technologies," *Eternal*, vol. 15, no. 2, pp. 378-387, Aug. 2024, doi: 10.26877/eternal.v15i2.830.

[35] M. Maqsood *et al*, "Assessment and Evaluation in Education 5.0:," in *Advances in Educational Technologies and Instructional Design*, A. Sorayyaei Azar, A. Albattat, M. Valeri, and V. Hassan, Eds, IGI Global, 2024, pp. 235-248. doi: 10.4018/979-8-3693-3041-8.ch013.

[36] P. Astuti, Y. N. Khairiyah, and W. A. Najwa, "EFEKTIVITAS ASSESMENT DIAGNOSTIK TERHADAP HASIL BELAJAR PESERTA DIDIK KELAS 2 SDI BAHRUL ULUM," *jpk*, vol. 5, no. 2, pp. 42-55, Jul. 2024, doi: 10.62426/jpk.v5i2.40.

[37] D. H. Alfageh, C. S. York, A. Hodge-Zickerman, and Y. Xie, "Elementary teachers' use of adaptive diagnostic assessment to improve mathematics teaching and learning: A case study," *INT ELECT J MATH ED*, vol. 19, no. 1, p. em0768, Feb. 2024, doi: 10.29333/iejme/14190.

[38] R. Theis, R. Junita, Kamid, and D. Iriani, "Diagnostic Tests Based on Three Level Tests on Fixed Materials for Students with Misconceptions," *j. pendidik. indonesia.* vol. 11, no. 4, Dec. 2022, doi: 10.23887/jpiundiksha.v11i4.50452.

[39] D. Nkomo and B. Dube, "Didactic Approaches to Inclusive Education Settings:," in *Advances in Educational Technologies and Instructional Design*, M. O. Maguvhe and M. M. Masuku, Eds, IGI Global, 2022, pp. 180-194. doi: 10.4018/978-1-6684-4436-8.ch014.

[40] T. Kärner, J. Warwas, and S. Schumann, "A Learning Analytics Approach to Address Heterogeneity in the Classroom: The Teachers' Diagnostic Support System," *Tech Know Learn*, vol. 26, no. 1, pp. 31-52, Mar. 2021, doi: 10.1007/s10758-020-09448-4.

[41] J. Thangaraj, "Formative Assessment as a Learning Method for Introductory Programming," in *Proceedings of the 2022 Conference on United Kingdom & Ireland Computing Education Research*, Dublin Ireland: ACM, Sep. 2022, pp. 1-2. doi: 10.1145/3555009.3555033.

[42] T. D. Wolsey and I. M. Karkouti, "Formative Assessment and Feedback for Language Learners," in *The TESOL Encyclopedia of English Language Teaching*, 1st ed, J. I. Liontas, T. International Association, and M. DelliCarpini, Eds, Wiley, 2024, pp. 1-9. doi: 10.1002/9781118784235.eelt1061.

[43] J. Qadir *et al*, "Leveraging the Force of Formative Assessment and Feedback for Effective Engineering Education," in *2020 ASEE Virtual Annual Conference Content Access Proceedings*, Virtual On line: ASEE Conferences, Jun. 2020, p. 34923. doi: 10.18260/1-2--34923.

[44] F. F. B. Pals, J. L. J. Tolboom, and C. J. M. Suhre, "Development of a formative assessment instrument to determine students' need for corrective actions in physics: Identifying students' functional level of understanding," *Thinking Skills and Creativity*, vol. 50, p. 101387, Dec. 2023, doi: 10.1016/j.tsc.2023.101387.

[45] B. Wisniewski and K. Zierer, "Functions and Success Conditions of Student Feedback in the Development of Teaching and Teachers," *in Student Feedback on Teaching in Schools*, W. Rollett, H. Bijlsma,

and S. Röhl, Eds. Röhl, Eds, Cham: Springer International Publishing, 2021, pp. 125-138. doi: 10.1007/978-3-030-75150-0_8.

[46] M. C. LoPresto, "Collaborative Learning and Formative Assessment in Astronomy," in *Active Learning in College Science*, J. J. Mintzes and E. M. Walter, Eds., Cham: Springer International Publishing, 2020, pp. 791-801. doi: 10.1007/978-3-030-33600-4_49.

[47] Q. M. J. Guillermo, S. Alberto Daniel, I. R. Ricardo Pedro, B. T. Juan Rolando, L. V. Rene Rafael, and M. C. J. Antonio, "Technological Tools in the Assessment of Meaningful Student Learning," *Intl. J. Rel.* vol. 5, no. 10, pp. 4732-4743, Jul. 2024, doi: 10.61707/cse01s14.

[48] E. Fani Prastikawati and . W., "Technology-based Formative Assessments Implemented by Secondary School English Teachers During Remote Learning," *KSS*, Sep. 2022, doi: 10.18502/kss.v7i14.11967.

[49] G. J. Cizek and S. N. Lim, "Formative assessment: an overview of history, theory and application," in *International Encyclopedia of Education(Fourth Edition)*, Elsevier, 2023, pp. 1-9. doi: 10.1016/B978-0-12-818630-5.09002-3.

[50] Y. Yang, "Formative Assessment: A Significant Facilitator of Student Learning," *Sci Insights Educ Front*, vol. 20, no. 2, pp. 3219-3221, Feb. 2024, doi: 10.15354/sief.24.co267.

[51] E. A. Tiana and N. Maruf, "Aligning Assessment and Curriculum: A Study of Summative Tests in Educational Settings," *JET ADI BUANA*, vol. 9, no. 01, pp. 29-36, Apr. 2024, doi: 10.36456/jet.v9.n01.2024.8884.

[52] I. De Florio, *From Assessment to Feedback: Applications in the Second/Foreign Language Classroom*, 1st ed. Cambridge University Press, 2023. doi: 10.1017/9781009218948.

[53] M. Leenknecht, L. Wijnia, M. Köhlen, L. Fryer, R. Rikers, and S. Loyens, "Formative assessment as practice: the role of students' motivation," *Assessment & Evaluation in Higher Education*, vol. 46, no. 2, pp. 236-255, Feb. 2021, doi: 10.1080/02602938.2020.1765228.

[54] B. Bloemen, W. Oortwijn, and G. J. Van Der Wilt, "Understanding the Normativity of Health Technology Assessment: Ontological, Moral, and Epistemological Commitments," *Health Care Anal*, Jun. 2024, doi: 10.1007/s10728-024-00487-x.

[55] M. N. Gaertner, "Norm-Referenced Assessment," in *Norm-Referenced Assessment*, Routledge, 2022. doi: 10.4324/9781138609877-REE13-1.

[56] E. Diaz-Bilello, "Criterion-Referenced Assessments," in *Criterion-Referenced Assessments*, Routledge, 2022. doi: 10.4324/9781138609877-REE10-1.

[57] P. Pui, B. Yuen, and H. Goh, "Using a criterion-referenced rubric to enhance student learning: a case study in a critical thinking and writing module," *Higher Education Research & Development*, vol. 40, no. 5, pp. 1056-1069, Jul. 2021, doi: 10.1080/07294360.2020.1795811.

[58] D. H. Murphy, J. L. Little, and E. L. Bjork, "The Value of Using Tests in Education as Tools for Learning-Not Just for Assessment," *Educ Psychol Rev*, vol. 35, no. 3, p. 89, Sep. 2023, doi: 10.1007/s10648-023-09808-3.

[59] Muhamad Ario Setiawan and Zaitun Qamariah, "A Practical Guide in Designing Curriculum for Diverse Learners," *PUSTAKA*, vol. 3, no. 3, pp. 260-275, Jul. 2023, doi: 10.56910/pustaka.v3i3.741.

[60] S. V. Rogatykh, "Practical works as a means of developing concepts of substances properties at an advanced level of studying chemistry in school," *Science and School*, no. 4, pp. 205-211, Aug. 2023, doi: 10.31862/1819-463X-2023-4-205-211.

[61]М. Москаленко and Л. Міронець, "Практичні роботи як засіб реалізації діяльнісного підходу під час навчання біології в старшій школі на профільному рівні," *naturalscience-vspu*, no. 6, pp. 9-16, Apr. 2024, doi: 10.31652/2786-5754-2024-6-9-16.

[62] N. M. Webb and E. Burnheimer, "Cooperative and collaborative learning," in *International Encyclopedia of Education(Fourth Edition)*, Elsevier, 2023, pp. 593-599. doi: 10.1016/B978-0-12-818630-5.14070-9.

[63] X. Shi, "Research on Project-based Learning in Practical English Education," *ER*, vol. 8, no. 3, pp. 433-437, Apr. 2024, doi: 10.26855/er.2024.03.017.

[64] S. A. Marley, A. Siani, and S. Sims, "Real-life research projects improve student engagement and provide reliable data for academics," *Ecology and Evolution*, vol. 12, no. 12, p. e9593, Dec. 2022, doi: 10.1002/ece3.9593.

[65] L. Pacursa, E. Alip, T. P. T. Do, and C. T. Trinh, "The art of classroom observation: The Case of Quirino State University and Can Tho University," *CTU J. of Inn. & Sus. Dev.* vol. 16, no. 2, pp. 105-115, Jul. 2024, doi: 10.22144/ctujoisd.2024.296.

[66] F. Tarusha and J. Bushi, "The Role of Classroom Observation, Its Impact on Improving Teacher's Teaching Practices," *ejtas*, vol. 2, no. 2, pp. 718-723, Mar. 2024, doi: 10.59324/ejtas.2024.2(2).63.

[67] P. Goble and R. C. Pianta, "Observation as a Lever for Teacher Improvement," in *Observation as a Lever for Teacher Improvement*, Routledge, 2022. doi: 10.4324/9781138609877-REE118-1.

[68] M. Lavadenz and E. G. Armas, *The Observation Protocol for Academic Literacies*. Multilingual Matters, 2024. doi: 10.21832/LAVADE9018.

[69] G. Asper, C. Faria, P. Serra, and C. Galvão, "Peer feedback and learning: a case study with 8th-grade Portuguese students," *Education 3-13*, pp. 1-18, Jul. 2024, doi: 10.1080/03004279.2024.2364610.

[70] Y. D. K. Sinaga, E. Arliani, J. C. Ngala, and N. L. I. T. Agustina, "Accuracy of Self-Assessment and Peer Assessment in Learning: A Systematic Literature Review," *j. paedagog. penelit. pengemb. pendidik.*, vol. 11, no. 2, p. 312, Apr. 2024, doi: 10.33394/jp.v11i2.9417.

[71] S. Wools, "All about validity: an evaluation system for the quality of educational assessment," University of Twente, 2015. doi: 10.3990/1.9789462597099.

[72] M. Liu and H. Yun, "Learning Goal Formulation Strategies in the Teaching-learning-assessment Alignment," *JEER*, vol. 9, no. 1, pp. 224-226, Jun. 2024, doi: 10.54097/eyr5s444.

[73] R. M. Teasdale, R. T. Pitts, E. F. Gates, and C. Shim, "Teaching specification of evaluative criteria: A guide for evaluation education," *New Drctns Evaluation*, vol. 2023, no. 177, pp. 31-37, Mar. 2023, doi: 10.1002/ev.20546.

[74] L. Nurlina and B. S. Wardianto, "Level of Validity towards the Development of Short Story Writing Teaching Materials for Class XI SMK in Banyumas Regency," in *Proceedings of the 1st International Conference of Humanities and Social Science, ICHSS 2021, 8 December 2021, Surakarta, Central Java, Indonesia*, Surakarta, Indonesia: EAI, 2022. doi: 10.4108/eai.8-12-2021.2322594.

[75] J. R. Korndorffer, "Principles of Validity," in *Comprehensive Healthcare Simulation: Surgery and Surgical Subspecialties*, D. Stefanidis, J. R. Korndorffer, and R. Sweet, Eds. in Comprehensive Healthcare Simulation. Cham: Springer International Publishing, 2019, pp. 37-39. doi: 10.1007/978-3-319-98276-2_4.

[76] K. Gupta, "Validity and Reliability of Students' Assessment: Case for Recognition as a Unified Concept of Valid Reliability," *International Journal of Applied & Basic Medical Research*, vol. 13, no. 3, pp. 129-132, Jul. 2023, doi: 10.4103/ijabmr.ijabmr_382_23.

[77] A. M. Haghighi, A. A. Kumar, and D. P. Mishev, "Reliability," in *Higher Mathematics for Science and Engineering*, Singapore: Springer Nature Singapore, 2024, pp. 545-583. doi: 10.1007/978-981-99-5431-5_9.

[78] D. Guzman-Orth, J. Steinberg, and T. Albee, "English learners who are blind or visually impaired: A participatory design approach to enhancing fairness and validity for language testing accommodations," *Language Testing*, vol. 40, no. 4, pp. 933-959, Oct. 2023, doi: 10.1177/02655322231159143.

[79] J. Tai, "Moving beyond reasonable adjustments: supporting employability through inclusive assessment design," *JTLGE*, vol. 14, no. 2, pp. 70-86, Oct. 2023, doi: 10.21153/jtlge2023vol14no2art1785.

[80] E. K. Vraga and S. Edgerly, "Relevance as a Mechanism in Evaluating News-Ness among American Teens and Adults," *Digital Journalism*, pp. 1-21, Sep. 2023, doi: 10.1080/21670811.2023.2250829.

[81] M. Mangla, V. Mehta, C. R. Pattnaik, and S. N. Mohanty, "Students' feedback- An effective tool toward enhancing the Teaching Learning Process," *ICST Transactions on Scalable Information Systems*, Jul. 2023, doi: 10.4108/eetsis.3347.

[82] F. A. P. Volpe, S. M. Quintana, M. D. C. Borges, and L. E. D. A. Troncon, "Avaliação do Estudante na Educação remota (ER) e à Distância (EAD): como desenvolver de modo efetivo, enfatizando a devolutiva," *Medicina (Ribeirão Preto)*, vol. 54, no. Supl 1, Aug. 2021, doi: 10.11606/issn.2176-7262.rmrp.2021.184773.

[83] K. Chatzistavrou, G. Kakarontzas, and L. Angelis, "Fuzzy Grading for Adaptability in a Learning Platform," in *Proceedings of the 20th Pan-Hellenic Conference on Informatics*, Patras Greece: ACM, Nov. 2016, pp. 1-4. doi: 10.1145/3003733.3003766.

[84] S. Elkington, "Shifts in Pedagogy and Flexible Assessment: Integrating Digital Technology with Good Teaching and Learning Practice," in *The Emerald Handbook of Higher Education in a Post-Covid World: New Approaches and Technologies for Teaching and Learning*, B. A. Brown and A. Irons, Eds., Emerald Publishing Limited, 2022, pp. 153-171. doi: 10.1108/978-1-80382-193-120221007.

[85] M. Polikoff, "Alignment," in *Alignment*, Routledge, 2022. doi: 10.4324/9781138609877-REE4-1.

[86] N. Bhaw and J. Kriek, "Using the Intended Curriculum's Prescribed Assessment Criteria to Measure Curriculum Assessment Alignment," Jun. 26, 2024. doi: 10.25159/UnisaRxiv/000086.v1.

[87] J. Norcini, "On Purpose: The Case for Alignment in Assessment," *Academic Medicine*, vol. 98, no. 11, pp. 1240-1242, Nov. 2023, doi: 10.1097/ACM.0000000000005430.

[88] M. Wilson, "Measuring progressions: Assessment structures underlying a learning progression," *J Res Sci Teach*, vol. 46, no. 6, pp. 716-730, Aug. 2009, doi: 10.1002/tea.20318.

[89] V. Thurner, A. Bottcher, and K. Schlierkamp, "Aligning learning objectives and exams: Moving upwards on the expertise level stack," in *2016 IEEE Global Engineering Education Conference*

(EDUCON), Abu Dhabi, United Arab Emirates: IEEE, Apr. 2016, pp. 455-462. doi: 10.1109/EDUCON.2016.7474593.
[90] R. M. Teasdale, "How Do You Define Success? Evaluative Criteria for Informal STEM Education," *Visitor Studies*, vol. 25, no. 2, pp. 163-184, Jul. 2022, doi: 10.1080/10645578.2022.2056397.
[91] N. Adamyan, "Scales for Assessing the Final Results of Various Forms of Student Learning," *Scientific Proceedings of Vanadzor State University: "Natural and Exact Sciences*, pp. 102-115, Jul. 2024, doi: 10.58726/27382923-ne2024.1-102.
[92] E. O. Bălănescu, "The Role of Learning Targets in Raising Student Achievement," *AUCSFLSA*, vol. 2024, no. 1, pp. 35-42, Jul. 2024, doi: 10.52744/AUCSFLSA.2024.01.05.
[93] D. K. Reed, "Clearly Communicating the Learning Objective Matters!: Clearly Communicating Lesson Objectives Supports Student Learning and Positive Behavior," *Middle School Journal*, vol. 43, no. 5, pp. 16-24, May 2012, doi: 10.1080/00940771.2012.11461825.
[94] N. Adamyan, "SAMPLE SCALE FOR ASSESSMENT OF THE FINAL RESULTS OF THE STUDENT'S PRACTICAL WORK," *SUSh Scientific Proceedings*, pp. 136-146, Dec. 2023, doi: 10.54151/27382559-23.2pb-136.
[95] L. Badenes-Ribera, N. C. Silver, and E. Pedroli, "Editorial: Scale Development and Score Validation," *Front. Psychol.* vol. 11, p. 799, Apr. 2020, doi: 10.3389/fpsyg.2020.00799.
[96] Center for Ethical Leadership, Karachi School of Business & Leadership (KSBL), Karachi. Pakistan. and F. Razzaq, "DOMINANT PRACTICES AND GUIDE FOR CREATING EFFECTIVE SURVEY SCALES IN SOCIAL SCIENCES," *pjsr*, vol. 04, no. 04, pp. 32-37, Dec. 2022, doi: 10.52567/pjsr.v4i04.785.
[97] C. M. Moss, "Learning Targets and Success Criteria," in *Learning Targets and Success Criteria*, Routledge, 2022. doi: 10.4324/9781138609877-REE39-1.
[98] C. S. Hartsough, K. D. Perez, and C. L. Swain, "Development and Scaling of a Preservice Teacher Rating Instrument," *Journal of*

Teacher Education, vol. 49, no. 2, pp. 132-139, Mar. 1998, doi: 10.1177/0022487198049002006.

[99] E. Wasserman and T. Ayeni, "Being Transparent about Assignment Expectations," in *Creating Culturally Affirming and Meaningful Assignments*, 1st ed. New York: Routledge, 2023, pp. 101-113. doi: 10.4324/9781003443797-8.

[100] L. P. Paudel, "Transparency in Course Assessments: A Robust Indicator of a Student-Centered Teaching," in *Advances in Educational Technologies and Instructional Design*, D. Akella, L. Paudel, N. Wickramage, M. Rogers, and A. Gibson, Eds., IGI Global, 2022, pp. 231-252. doi: 10.4018/978-1-7998-9549-7.ch011.

[101] J. Cherniavsky and E. Hamilton, "The Learning Grid," in *Computer Support for Collaborative Learning*, 1st ed. New York: Routledge, 2023, pp. 733-734. doi: 10.4324/9781315045467-196.

[102] Kuban State Agrarian University named after I.T. Trubilin *et al*, "Multi-criteria system for evaluating students," *Alma mater (Moskva)*, no. 4, pp. 54-58, Apr. 2023, doi: 10.20339/AM.04-23.054.

[103] F. Ndaji and P. Tymms, "The P scales: how well are they working?," *British J Special Edu*, vol. 37, no. 4, pp. 198-208, Dec. 2010, doi: 10.1111/j.1467-8578.2010.00481.x.

[104] H. Oliveira and J. Bonito, "Practical work in science education: a systematic literature review," *Front. Educ.* vol. 8, pp. 1151641, May 2023, doi: 10.3389/feduc.2023.1151641.

[105] Zaker Ul Oman, Sumeet Pandey, and Ashitosh Gaddam, "A study on impact of conceptual and practical based learning on employability," *World J. Adv. Res. Rev.*, vol. 16, no. 2, pp. 486-492, Nov. 2022, doi: 10.30574/wjarr.2022.16.2.1204.

[106] G. O. Martin-Kniep, "Performance Assessment," in *Performance Assessment*, Routledge, 2022. doi: 10.4324/9781138609877-REE151-1.

[107] B. T. Drumm, R. Bree, C. S. Griffin, and N. O'Leary, "Diversifying laboratory assessment modes broadens engagement with practical competencies in life science students," *Advances in Physiology Education*, vol. 48, no. 3, pp. 527-546, Sep. 2024, doi: 10.1152/advan.00257.2023.

[108] "Role of Simulation-Based Learning in Skill Development of Students: An Empirical Study in Context of ICT-Driven Education World," *Journal of Informatics Education and Research*, 2024, doi: 10.52783/jier.v4i2.1117.

[109] D. I. Cajamarca Carrazco, D. P. Hidalgo Cajo, J. A. Jhon Alexander Ponce Alencastro, and N. Típula Quispe, "Evaluation of the use of virtual simulators for training in problem-solving skills in university students," *Salud, Ciencia y Tecnología*, vol. 4, p. 1281, Jan. 2024, doi: 10.56294/saludcyt20241281.

[110] M. K. Wang and D. Brandt Vegas, "Direct Observation and Feedback on the Internal Medicine Clinical Teaching Unit," *Can Journ Gen Int Med*, vol. 17, no. 4, pp. 48-58, Nov. 2022, doi: 10.22374/cjgim.v17i4.635.

[111] M. Das, N. K. Das, I. Mohapatra, and S. Sen, "Effectiveness of demonstration, observation, assistance, and performance sessions in imparting visual assessment skills to phase 3 medical students," *International Journal of Academic Medicine*, vol. 9, no. 4, pp. 192-200, Oct. 2023, doi: 10.4103/ijam.ijam_26_23.

[112] P. Eidesen, A. Bjune, and S. Lang, "'Show me how to use a microscope' - The development and evaluation of certification as direct assessment of practical lab skills," Mar. 06, 2023, *Preprints*. doi: 10.22541/au.167813479.91520887/v1.

[113] Z. Barends, A. Lebethe, and A. H. M. Jacobs, "Portfolios as assessment for learning: A case study of pre-service Foundation Phase teacher education students," *SAJHE*, vol. 37, no. 2, 2023, doi: 10.20853/37-2-5403.

[114] Nurhayani, M. Botifar, and D. Wanto, "Portfolio Assessment in Scope of Learning Competence-Based Islamic Religious Education (PAI)," *JEDA*, vol. 2, no. 1, pp. 21-34, Feb. 2023, doi: 10.55927/jeda.v2i1.1939.

[115] D. Fanelli, "A theory and methodology to quantify knowledge," *R. Soc. open sci.* vol. 6, no. 4, p. 181055, Apr. 2019, doi: 10.1098/rsos.181055.

[116] M. Paniagua, K. A. Swygert, and S. M. Downing, "Written Tests: Writing High-Quality Constructed-Response and Selected-

Response Items," in *Assessment in Health Professions Education*, 2nd ed., R. Yudkowsky, Y. S. Park, and S. M. Downing, Eds., Routledge, 2019, pp. 109-126. doi: 10.4324/9781315166902-7.

[117] V. Villarroel, D. Boud, S. Bloxham, D. Bruna, and C. Bruna, "Using principles of authentic assessment to redesign written examinations and tests," *Innovations in Education and Teaching International*, vol. 57, no. 1, pp. 38-49, Jan. 2020, doi: 10.1080/14703297.2018.1564882.

[118] R. Əliyev, "21st CENTURY SKILLS IN EDUCATION: OUR YESTERDAY, TODAY," *SW*, vol. 91, no. 3, pp. 31-36, Aug. 2024, doi: 10.69682/azrt.2024.91(3).31-36.

[119] M. U. Tariq, "Enhancing Students and Learning Achievement as 21st-Century Skills Through Transdisciplinary Approaches:," in *Advances in Higher Education and Professional Development*, R. Kumar, E. T. Ong, S. Anggoro, and T. L. Toh, Eds, IGI Global, 2024, pp. 220-257. doi: 10.4018/979-8-3693-3699-1.ch007.

[120] T. Otarova, M. Assylbekova, B. Batanassova, S. Abdrakhman, and Z. Koshimbetova, "The level of formation of Transversal competence in the context of higher education: The case of Kazakhstan," *Ias*, no. 56, pp. 1908-1915, Apr. 2024, doi: 10.54919/physics/56.2024.190tr8.

[121] O. Rojas and S. Pech, "CRITICAL THINKING AS A TRANSVERSAL COMPETENCE IN HIGH SCHOOL STUDENTS: ANALYSIS OF THE PSYCHOMETRIC PROPERTIES OF A COMPETENCY MEASUREMENT INSTRUMENT," presented at the 16th annual International Conference of Education, Research and Innovation, Seville, Spain, Nov. 2023, pp. 9025-9033. doi: 10.21125/iceri.2023.2300.

[122] D. Naqia, A. As'ari, and A. Suaidi, "Students' Critical Thinking Skills Perform in Debate Activities," *JELTS*, vol. 6, no. 1, pp. 55-64, Mar. 2023, doi: 10.48181/jelts.v6i1.17491.

[123] D. A. Dewangga, I. Rosadi, N. M. Muna, and L. Indriani, "Investigating Critical Thinking Skills in Debate Class through the Use of the Case Method," *Pedagogy: Jour. of. Eng. Lang. Teach*, vol. 12, no. 1, p. 117, Jun. 2024, doi: 10.32332/joelt.v12i1.9266.

[124] M. M. Modak, P. Gharpure, and S. M, "Adaptive Learning and Correlative Assessment of Differential Usage Patterns for Students with-or-without Learning Disabilities via Learning Analytics," *ACM Trans. Asian Low-Resour. Lang. Inf. Process.* vol. 22, no. 12, pp. 1-25, Dec. 2023, doi: 10.1145/3632365.

[125] R. D. K. Wardhani, "Education and Learning Services for Children with Learning Difficulties The Child With Special Needed," *sssh*, vol. 2, no. 2, pp. 125-131, May 2023, doi: 10.51773/sssh.v2i2.242.

[126] "Innovative tools for the direct assessment of social and emotional skills," OECD Education Working Papers 316, Jun. 2024. doi: 10.1787/eed9bb04-en.

[127] C. M. Onumah *et al*, "Strategies for Advancing Equity in Frontline Clinical Assessment," *Academic Medicine*, vol. 98, no. 8S, pp. S57-S63, Aug. 2023, doi: 10.1097/ACM.0000000000005246.

[128] K. R. Moore, T. R. Amidon, and M. Simmons, "Equity and Inclusion as Workplace Practices: A Four-Step Process for Moving to Action," *tech. comm.*, vol. 70, no. 3, pp. 7-27, Aug. 2023, doi: 10.55177/tc710097.

[129] Q. Ma, "The Investigation of the Test Accommodations for Students with Disabilities," *LNEP*, vol. 35, no. 1, pp. 289-294, Jan. 2024, doi: 10.54254/2753-7048/35/20232149.

[130] A. S. Hapsara, "Evaluasi Pelaksanaan Akomodasi Kurikulum untuk Peserta Didik dengan Hambatan Penglihatan pada Pelajaran Sosiologi," *ideguru*, vol. 9, no. 1, pp. 46-55, Nov. 2023, doi: 10.51169/ideguru.v9i1.761.

[131] Y. K. Nurlankyzy, B. Adilkhanova, and M. Zhunissova, "Adapting Assessment Tools: Teachers' Perceptions on the Integration of AI Tools in Student Homework Assignments," *INTERNATIONAL ADVANCED RESEARCH JOURNAL IN SCIENCE, ENGINEERING AND TECHNOLOGY*, vol. 11, no. 5, Apr. 2024, doi: 10.17148/IARJSET.2024.11511.

[132] A. A. Molina-Moreira, O. J. Velásquez-Orellana, D. J. Zambrano-Murillo, and M. E. Zambrano-Villamil, "Importance of feedback in the student evaluation process," *ijss*, vol. 6, no. 3, pp. 168-172, Jul. 2023, doi: 10.21744/ijss.v6n3.2176.

[133] R. Rajapakse, "The Impact of Feedback on the Progress of Teaching Learning Process and the Overall Student Performance," Jun. 18, 2024, *Open Science Framework*. doi: 10.31219/osf.io/suqz5.

[134] D. Carless, "Feedback for student learning in higher education," in *International Encyclopedia of Education(Fourth Edition)*, Elsevier, 2023, pp. 623-629. doi: 10.1016/B978-0-12-818630-5.14066-7.

[135] Tashkent State University of Uzbek Language and Literature Faculty of Translation Theory and Practice, D. Ermanov, Z. Ergasheva. Ergasheva, and Tashkent State University of Uzbek Language and Literature Faculty of Translation Theory and Practice, "MAKING ASSESSMENT AND CONSTRUCTIVE FEEDBACK," in *Modern approaches and new trends in teaching foreign languages*, Alisher Navo'i Tashkent state university of Uzbek language and literature, May 2024, pp. 68-83. doi: 10.52773/tsuull.conf.teach.foreign.lang.2024.8.5/HTPT6600.

[136] . Asnawi and . Wariyati, "The impact of using feedback to increase students' motivation at the University of Muslim Nusantara Al Washliyah Medan," *RSD*, vol. 10, no. 1, p. e38210111784, Jan. 2021, doi: 10.33448/rsd-v10i1.11784.

[137] E. Illarionova, "STUDYING THE INFLUENCE OF FEEDBACK ON MOTIVATION AND PERFORMANCE RESULTS," *Management of the Personnel and Intellectual Resources in Russia*, vol. 13, no. 2, pp. 10-12, Jun. 2024, doi: 10.12737/2305-7807-2024-13-2-10-12.

[138] C. Li, Z. Yang, and Y. Yang, "The Impact of Peer Feedback on Student Learning Effectiveness: A Meta-analysis Based on 39 Experimental or Quasiexperimental Studies," in *Computer Science and Educational Informatization*, vol. 1899, J. Gan, Y. Pan, J. Zhou, D. Liu, X. Song, and Z. Lu, Eds. in Communications in Computer and Information Science, vol. 1899. Singapore: Springer Nature Singapore, 2024, pp. 42-52. doi: 10.1007/978-981-99-9499-1_4.

[139] H. C. Khoza, "Dialogue with Students as a Valuable Tool in Teacher Inquiry for Professional Development: A narrative of a novice science teacher educator learning about student interaction in biology classrooms," *JoSoTL*, vol. 24, no. 1, Mar. 2024, doi: 10.14434/josotl.v24i1.35486.

[140] R. E. Stup, "Giving and receiving feedback," *AABP Proceedings*, no. 55, pp. 142-144, Jul. 2023, doi: 10.21423/aabppro20228630.
[141] A. Díaz-Vicario, M. D. M. Duran-Bellonch, and G. Ion, "Contribution of peer-feedback to the development of teamwork skills," *Active Learning in Higher Education*, p. 14697874241238758, Mar. 2024, doi: 10.1177/14697874241238758.
[142] B. Rassameethes, K. Phusavat, Z. Pastuszak, A. N. Hidayanto, and J. Majava, "Constructive feedback and the perceived impacts on learning and development by the learners' genders," *HSM*, vol. 42, no. 5, pp. 487-498, Sep. 2023, doi: 10.3233/HSM-220172.
[143] K. Leka and D. Beshiri, "School leaders' and teachers' perceptions of the feedback and evaluation system in Albania," *61*, vol. 12, no. 3, pp. 1054-1067, Jul. 2024, doi: 10.18488/61.v12i3.3823.
[144] E. A. Dolan, B. L. Fleming, D. P. Keppel, and J. M. Covert, "Sandwich With a Side of Motivation: An Investigation of the Effects of the Feedback Sandwich Method on Motivation," presented at the The IAFOR International Conference on Education - Hawaii 2022, Mar. 2022, pp. 297-306. doi: 10.22492/issn.2189-1036.2022.28.
[145] R. K. M.R, "Teacher-Student Feedback Dynamics And Their Implications For Effective Teaching," *EATP*, pp. 9671-9677, May 2024, doi: 10.53555/kuey.v30i5.4636.
[146] "Preferred Methods of Providing Critique to Students and Teachers in the English Language Classroom," *Inf. Sci. Lett.* vol. 12, no. 9, pp. 2199-2210, Sep. 2023, doi: 10.18576/isl/120925.
[147] K. M. O'Brien, M. M. Cumming, G. D. Binkert, and D. R. Oré, "Providing Positive and Constructive Feedback," in *High Leverage Practices for Inclusive Classrooms*, 2nd ed. New York: Routledge, 2022, pp. 343-356. doi: 10.4324/9781003148609-28.
[148] K. Eriksson, J. Lindvall, O. Helenius, and A. Ryve, "Cultural Variation in the Effectiveness of Feedback on Students' Mistakes," *Front. Psychol.* vol. 10, p. 3053, Jan. 2020, doi: 10.3389/fpsyg.2019.03053.
[149] L. E. Aznar-Mas, L. Atarés Huerta, and J. A. Marin-Garcia, "Effectiveness of the use of open-ended questions in student evaluation of teaching in an engineering degree," *JIEM*, vol. 16, no. 3, p. 521, Oct. 2023, doi: 10.3926/jiem.5620.

[150] M. Small, "The Power of Open-Ended Questions," *Mathematics Teacher: Learning and Teaching PK-12*, vol. 117, no. 7, pp. 528-529, Jul. 2024, doi: 10.5951/MTLT.2024.0050.

[151] X. Lu, W. Wang, B. A. Motz, W. Ye, and N. T. Heffernan, "Immediate text-based feedback timing on foreign language online assignments: How immediate should immediate feedback be?," *Computers and Education Open*, vol. 5, pp. 100148, Dec. 2023, doi: 10.1016/j.caeo.2023.100148.

[152] L.-C. Durán-Terrádez and T. Baviera, "Speaking without Hurting: Assertiveness and Psychological Safety in Receiving Criticism," *Revista Empresa y Humanismo*, pp. 9-32, Jun. 2023, doi: 10.15581/015.XXVI.2.9-32.

[153] J. Hu and Y. Zhang, "Growth mindset mediates perceptions of teachers' and parents' process feedback in digital reading performance: Evidence from 32 OECD countries," *Learning and Instruction*, vol. 90, p. 101874, Apr. 2024, doi: 10.1016/j.learninstruc.2024.101874.

[154] T. Zhang, "Study of Parent-Teacher Interactions of Improving Student Achievement," *BCPSSH*, vol. 17, pp. 177-183, May 2022, doi: 10.54691/bcpssh.v17i.641.

[155] Y. Lu and E. Sarmiento, "Research on the Comprehensive Quality Improvement of College Students through School-family Collaborative Education," *JEER*, vol. 9, no. 1, pp. 292-295, Jun. 2024, doi: 10.54097/sr57k232.

[156] S. A. Nagro, "PROSE Checklist: Strategies for Improving School-to-Home Written Communication," *TEACHING Exceptional Children*, vol. 47, no. 5, pp. 256-263, May 2015, doi: 10.1177/0040059915580031.

[157] E. Perego, *Accessible Communication: A Cross-country Journey*. Frank & Timme, 2020. doi: 10.26530/20.500.12657/50590.

[158] M. N. Velasco *et al*, "Enhancing Parent-Teacher Collaboration in Early Childhood Education through a Web-Based App," in *2024 7th International Conference on Informatics and Computational Sciences (ICICoS)*, Semarang, Indonesia: IEEE, Jul. 2024, pp. 131-136. doi: 10.1109/ICICoS62600.2024.10636878.

[159] E. Munthe and E. Westergård, "Parents', teachers', and students' roles in parent-teacher conferences; a systematic review and meta-synthesis," *Teaching and Teacher Education*, vol. 136, p. 104355, Dec. 2023, doi: 10.1016/j.tate.2023.104355.

[160] L. Aust, B. Schütze, J. Hochweber, and E. Souvignier, "Effects of formative assessment on intrinsic motivation in primary school mathematics instruction," *Eur J Psychol Educ*, vol. 39, no. 3, pp. 2177-2200, Sep. 2024, doi: 10.1007/s10212-023-00768-4.

[161] R. A. Kusurkar *et al*, "The Effect of Assessments on Student Motivation for Learning and Its Outcomes in Health Professions Education: A Review and Realist Synthesis," *Academic Medicine*, vol. 98, no. 9, pp. 1083-1092, Sep. 2023, doi: 10.1097/ACM.0000000000005263.

[162] A. Nazish and M. A. Kang, "Exploring the Positive Teacher-Student Relationship on Students' Motivation and Academic Performance in Secondary Schools in Karachi," *AESSR*, vol. 4, no. 2, pp. 149-159, May 2024, doi: 10.48112/aessr.v4i2.710.

[163] A. Afrilia, "THE IMPACT OF TEACHER-STUDENTS RELATIONSHIP ON ENGLISH STUDENTS' MOTIVATION (A SURVEY ON THE FIRST YEAR ENGLISH DEPARTMENT STUDENTS)," *JP*, no. Volume 09 No. 2 Juni 2024, Jun. 2024, doi: 10.23969/jp.v9i2.13651.

[164] D. Tila and D. Levy, "Increasing Students' Growth Mindset and Learning Perception by Allowing Online Revision and Resubmission in a Community College," *SER*, pp. 23-38, Dec. 2023, doi: 10.37256/ser.5120243499.

[165] J. Zhang, Y. Liu, and C. M. Cheong, "The effect of growth mindset on motivation and strategy use in Hong Kong students' integrated writing performance," *Eur J Psychol Educ*, vol. 39, no. 3, pp. 2915-2934, Sep. 2024, doi: 10.1007/s10212-024-00859-w.

[166] G. B. Amangeldina and D. L. Dudovich, "The impact of pedagogical assessment on increasing motivation to learn and the quality of education," *FLER*, vol. 3, no. 1, pp. 11-23, Sep. 2022, doi: 10.35213/2686-7516-2022-3-1-11-23.

[167] P. A. Schutz, "Where Will Michelle Go to College? Culture and Context in the Study of Motivation," in *Motivation Science*, 1st ed,

M. Bong, J. Reeve, and S. Kim, Eds, Oxford University PressNew York, 2023, pp. 83-87. doi: 10.1093/oso/9780197662359.003.0014.

[168] K. R. Wentzel, "Improving Social Contexts Can Enhance Student Motivation," in *Motivation Science*, 1st ed, M. Bong, J. Reeve, and S. Kim, Eds, Oxford University PressNew York, 2023, pp. 350-355. doi: 10.1093/oso/9780197662359.003.0058.

[169] M. Keumala, N. M. Samad, I. A. Samad, and N. Rachmawaty, "THE INFLUENCE OF SOCIO CULTURAL AND EDUCATIONAL BACKGROUND ON EFL LEARNERS' MOTIVATION," *ITJ*, vol. 1, no. 1, pp. 67-77, Mar. 2019, doi: 10.24256/itj.v1i1.556.

[170] V. Tamášová, A. Lobotková, and I. Marks, "MOTIVATION OF TEACHERS AND STUDENTS AS PART OF FORMATIVE EDUCATION," *AD ALTA: Journal of Interdisciplinary Research*, vol. 14, no. 1, pp. 252-260, Jun. 2024, doi: 10.33543/j.1401.252260.

[171] K. K. S. Chan, "Section Overview," in *The Routledge International Handbook of Life and Values Education in Asia*, 1st ed., London: Routledge, 2024, pp. 313-316. doi: 10.4324/9781003352471-40.

[172] M. Hung, "Goal-Setting Displayed by Vietnamese EFL Students," Apr. 26, 2023, *SocArXiv*. doi: 10.31235/osf.io/kfnuv.

[173] "Gheorghe Asachi" Technical University, Iasi, Romania, O. Jitaru, R. Axinte, and C. Vatavu, "THE ROLE OF PERSONAL DEVELOPMENT IN STUDENTS ADAPTING TO THE ACADEMIC LIFE," in *SCIENTIFIC RESEARCH AND EDUCATION IN THE AIR FORCE*, Publishing House of "Henri Coanda" Air Force Academy, Feb. 2022, pp. 63-70. doi: 10.19062/2247-3173.2021.22.10.

[174] "An Assessment on Growth of Knowledge and Skills," *cellrm*, vol. 2, no. 2, pp. 31-38, Jul. 2023, doi: 10.46632/cellrm/2/2/4.

[175] M. M. Wadi, M. S. B. Yusoff, M. H. Taha, S. Shorbagi, N. A. Z. Nik Lah, and A. F. Abdul Rahim, "The framework of Systematic Assessment for Resilience (SAR): development and validation," *BMC Med Educ*, vol. 23, no. 1, p. 213, Apr. 2023, doi: 10.1186/s12909-023-04177-5.

[176] T. H. Yong, "The A-B-C of Engaging Students With Feedback to Build Resilient Learners," presented at The Asian Conference on

Education 2022, Feb. 2023, pp. 101-115. doi: 10.22492/issn.2186-5892.2023.8.

[177] S. Romadlan, D. Wahdiyati, H. Prasetya, and R. N. Sari, "Building Interpersonal Communication Skills in the Digital Age for Vocational Students in South Jakarta," *PRO*, vol. 6, no. 6, pp. 702-707, Dec. 2023, doi: 10.32832/pro.v6i6.510.

[178] Novosibirsk State Pedagogical University, N. N. Zhuravleva, V. G. Yaroslavtsev, and Novosibirsk State University of Economics and Management, "Methods for Assessing the Personal Results of Mastering the Main Educational Program as a Component of Students' Self-Development," *Journal of Pedagogical Innovations*, no. 2, pp. 36-46, Jul. 2023, doi: 10.15293/1812-9463.2302.04.

[179] J. Burton and N. Jackson, "Roles of self-assessment tools and work-based learning in personal development," in *Assessment in Medical Education and Training*, 1st ed., London: CRC Press, 2023, pp. 131-139. doi: 10.1201/9781846197994-12.

[180] C. Bosch, "Assessing the psychometric properties of the intrinsic motivation inventory in blended learning environments," *JEELR*, vol. 11, no. 2, pp. 263-271, Mar. 2024, doi: 10.20448/jeelr.v11i2.5468.

[181] W. J. Arcegono *et al*, "The Connection Between Teachers' Mindsets and Methods of Assessment in the Classroom," *JGI*, vol. 2, no. 03, pp. 146-154, Oct. 2023, doi: 10.56741/jgi.v2i03.441.

[182] F. Al Husseiny, "Assessment in the Digital Age:," in *Advances in Educational Marketing, Administration, and Leadership*, F. Al Husseiny and A. S. Munna, Eds., IGI Global, 2024, pp. 47-69. doi: 10.4018/979-8-3693-1536-1.ch003.

[183] L. Isak, O. Babak, and Y. Hren, "Digital Tools in Professional Education Training," *PEMTT*, no. 18, pp. 104-125, Dec. 2023, doi: 10.31470/2415-3729-2023-18-104-125.

[184] Rohini Unnikrishnan, "Digital Integration: A Productive Pedagogy and its Efficacy of Language Learning," *rtdh*, vol. 12, no. S1-Dec, pp. 229-234, Dec. 2023, doi: 10.34293/rtdh.v12iS1-Dec.114.

[185] R. Lam, "E-Portfolios for self-regulated and co-regulated learning: A review," *Front. Psychol.* vol. 13, p. 1079385, Nov. 2022, doi: 10.3389/fpsyg.2022.1079385.

[186] S. Yadav, "Designing Effective E-Portfolios for Authentic Assessment: Encouraging Reflection and Promoting Student Ownership," in *Advances in Educational Technologies and Instructional Design*, L. Marron, Ed., IGI Global, 2024, pp. 235-258. doi: 10.4018/979-8-3693-1001-4.ch011.

[187] A. S. Mawela, M. M. Van Wyk, and J. Dreyer, "The Use of Technology to Enhance the High-Quality Assessment of E-Portfolios in Institutions of Higher Learning:," in *Advances in Educational Technologies and Instructional Design*, C. E. M. Tabane, B. M. Diale, A. S. Mawela, and T. V. Zengele, Eds, IGI Global, 2023, pp. 229-253. doi: 10.4018/978-1-6684-6995-8.ch013.

[188] E. Walland and S. Shaw, "E-portfolios in teaching, learning and assessment: tensions in theory and praxis," *Technology, Pedagogy and Education*, vol. 31, no. 3, pp. 363-379, May 2022, doi: 10.1080/1475939X.2022.2074087.

[189] A. K. Abdallah, M. H. Aljanahi, and H. A. Almejalli, "The Power of Peer Review: Harnessing Collaborative Insights for Authentic Assessment," in *Advances in Educational Technologies and Instructional Design*, A. K. Abdallah, A. M. Alkaabi, and R. Al-Riyami, Eds, IGI Global, 2024, pp. 232-247. doi: 10.4018/979-8-3693-0880-6.ch016.

[190] B. D. A. Aprilianti and A. Widyantoro, "Digital Peer Feedback and Students' Critical Thinking: What Correlation and to What Extent?," *JOLLT*, vol. 12, no. 2, p. 629, Apr. 2024, doi: 10.33394/jollt.v12i2.10264.

[191] G. V. Helden, V. Van Der Werf, G. N. Saunders-Smits, and M. M. Specht, "The Use of Digital Peer Assessment in Higher Education-An Umbrella Review of Literature," *IEEE Access*, vol. 11, pp. 22948-22960, 2023, doi: 10.1109/ACCESS.2023.3252914.

[192] S. A. Burr *et al*, "A narrative review of adaptive testing and its application to medical education," *MedEdPublish*, vol. 13, p. 221, Oct. 2023, doi: 10.12688/mep.19844.1.

[193] M. Shafique, A. F. Fazli, L. Qureshi, and W. Saleem, "Adaptive Learning for Standardized Test Preparation," in *2023 25th International Multitopic Conference (INMIC)*, Lahore, Pakistan: IEEE, Nov. 2023, pp. 1-8. doi: 10.1109/INMIC60434.2023.10465975.

[194] K. Éva, E. Nagy, and G. Molnár, "Adaptive ICT-based evaluation system in teaching and learning process," in *2023 IEEE 27th International Conference on Intelligent Engineering Systems (INES)*, Nairobi, Kenya: IEEE, Jul. 2023, pp. 000089-000094. doi: 10.1109/INES59282.2023.10297735.

[195] P. Kannan and D. Zapata-Rivera, "Facilitating the Use of Data From Multiple Sources for Formative Learning in the Context of Digital Assessments: Informing the Design and Development of Learning Analytic Dashboards," *Front. Educ.* vol. 7, p. 913594, Jun. 2022, doi: 10.3389/feduc.2022.913594.

[196] D. Amo-Filva, B. D. Beby, F. J. Garcia-Penalvo, and J. Chen, "Towards an ethical data literacy proficiency: a Moodle logs analytical tool," in *2022 XII International Conference on Virtual Campus (JICV)*, Arequipa, Peru: IEEE, Sep. 2022, pp. 1-3. doi: 10.1109/JICV56113.2022.9934790.

[197] M. Q. Ramadhan and N. L. Inayati, "Benefits of Digital Tools in Learning Evaluation," *jupenus*, vol. 2, no. 1, pp. 91-96, Jun. 2024, doi: 10.59996/jurnalpelitanusantara.v2i1.348.

[198] L. Serutla, A. Mwanza, and T. Celik, "Online Assessments in a Changing Education Landscape," in *Reimagining Education - The Role of E-Learning, Creativity, and Technology in the Post-Pandemic Era*, S. Mistretta, Ed., IntechOpen, 2024. doi: 10.5772/intechopen.1002176.

[199] A. Najar, A. E. Moutaouaki, and M. A. Ahmed, "Course Learning Outcomes Evaluation Through Online Assignments," *BJMAS*, vol. 5, no. 4, pp. 1-7, Jul. 2024, doi: 10.37745/bjmas.2022.04136.

[200] H. Yildiz and S. I. Kuru Gonen, "AUTOMATED WRITING EVALUATION SYSTEM FOR FEEDBACK IN THE DIGITAL WORLD: AN ONLINE LEARNING OPPORTUNITY FOR ENGLISH AS A FOREIGN LANGUAGE STUDENTS," *Turkish Online Journal of Distance Education*, vol. 25, no. 3, pp. 183-206, Jul. 2024, doi: 10.17718/tojde.1169727.

[201] X. Yuan, "The Impact of Automated Evaluation Feedback on Students' Writing Revision," *IJLLL*, vol. 9, no. 4, pp. 526-529, Dec. 2023, doi: 10.18178/IJLLL.2023.9.6.464.

[202] M. Skála, "Benefits and Pitfalls of Electronic Knowledge Testing," *ACC JOURNAL*, vol. 29, no. 3, pp. 116-123, Dec. 2023, doi: 10.2478/acc-2023-0019.

[203] N. V. Hausmann-Ushkova, O. E. Shults, and G. M. Pervova, "Providing students with feedback during online language projects," *jour*, vol. 29, no. 2, pp. 337-348, Apr. 2024, doi: 10.20310/1810-0201-2024-29-2-337-348.

[204] A. Stanoyevitch, "Online assessment in the age of artificial intelligence," *Discov Educ*, vol. 3, no. 1, p. 126, Aug. 2024, doi: 10.1007/s44217-024-00212-9.

[205] R. Sultana, R. Mollika, A. K. Sumy, S. Shahjamal, F. Alam, and P. Ashraf, "Benefits and Challenges of Online Teaching Learning from the Students' View," *Delta Med Col J*, vol. 9, no. 2, pp. 69-74, Jul. 2024, doi: 10.3329/dmcj.v9i2.74868.

[206] H. J. Agtarap, A. C. Januto, K. A. Aglibot, and C. M. Toquero, "Assessment strategies and challenges of teachers in evaluating students during online learning," *Journal of Digital Educational Technology*, vol. 4, no. 2, p. ep2418, Jul. 2024, doi: 10.30935/jdet/14863.

[207] K. Jalilzadeh, M. Rashtchi, and F. Mirzapour, "Cheating in online assessment: a qualitative study on reasons and coping strategies focusing on EFL teachers' perceptions," *Lang Test Asia*, vol. 14, no. 1, p. 29, Jul. 2024, doi: 10.1186/s40468-024-00304-1.

[208] N. Taşkın, "Cheating and Prevention Strategies in Online Assessment:," in *Advances in Educational Marketing, Administration, and Leadership*, G. Chemsi, I. Elimadi, M. Sadiq, and M. Radid, Eds., IGI Global, 2024, pp. 151-172. doi: 10.4018/979-8-3693-3045-6.ch009.

[209] M. Djalalov, "Digital Challenges in Education," *Uzbek J. Law Digi. Policy*, vol. 2, no. 2, Oct. 2023, doi: 10.59022/ujldp.127.

[210] M. D. C. Da Costa, A. L. S. Olinda, and A. P. Dos Santos, "Digital technologies in education: Challenges and opportunities for

teaching and learning," in *VI Seven International Multidisciplinary Congress*, Seven Congress, Jul. 2024. doi: 10.56238/sevenVImulti2024-019.

[211] J. Humphries, K. Carroll, and J. Varkey, "The Importance of Data in Teaching and Learning," in *Work-Integrated Learning Case Studies in Teacher Education*, M. Winslade, T. Loughland, and M. J. Eady, Eds., Singapore: Springer Nature Singapore, 2023, pp. 147-155. doi: 10.1007/978-981-19-6532-6_12.

[212] G. S. Maxwell, "Different Approaches to Data Use," in *Using Data to Improve Student Learning*, vol. 9, in The Enabling Power of Assessment, vol. 9. Cham: Springer International Publishing, 2021, pp. 11-71. doi: 10.1007/978-3-030-63539-8_2.

[213] K. Rekha, K. Gopal, D. Satheeskumar, U. A. Anand, D. S. S. Doss, and S. Elayaperumal, "Ai-Powered Personalized Learning System Design: Student Engagement And Performance Tracking System," in *2024 4th International Conference on Advance Computing and Innovative Technologies in Engineering (ICACITE)*, Greater Noida, India: IEEE, May 2024, pp. 1125-1130. doi: 10.1109/ICACITE60783.2024.10617155.

[214] K. Kaur and O. Dahiya, "Role of Educational Data Mining and Learning Analytics Techniques Used for Predictive Modeling," in *2023 3rd International Conference on Innovative Practices in Technology and Management (ICIPTM)*, Uttar Pradesh, India: IEEE, Feb. 2023, pp. 1-6. doi: 10.1109/ICIPTM57143.2023.10117779.

[215] N. Shirisha, G. Divyajyothi, A. Prashanthi, and G. Sowmya, "Student Data Analysis using Hadoop," in *2023 7th International Conference on Intelligent Computing and Control Systems (ICICCS)*, Madurai, India: IEEE, May 2023, pp. 1092-1096. doi: 10.1109/ICICCS56967.2023.10142250.

[216] J. A. L. Rodríguez, N. D. Díaz, and C. D. B. González, "Optimizing Education with Data Analytics: A Feature Comparison of LMS and SIS," May 08, 2024, *Computer Science and Mathematics*. doi: 10.20944/preprints202405.0459.v1.

[217] J. Novák, "Evaluation of Student Feedback as a Tool for Higher Education Quality Enhancement," *R&E-SOURCE*, pp. 117-127, Jun. 2023, doi: 10.53349/resource.2023.is1.a1196.

[218] M. Karvonen, L. Ruhter, and A. K. Clark, "Data to Inform Academic Instruction for Students with Extensive Support Needs: Availability, Use, and Perceptions," *Exceptionality*, vol. 32, no. 3, pp. 183-202, May 2024, doi: 10.1080/09362835.2024.2313748.

[219] D. Heyne, G. A. Keppens, and D. Dvořák, "From Attendance Data to Student Support: International Practices for Recording, Reporting, and Using Data on School Attendance and Absence," *ORBIS SCHOLAE*, vol. 16, no. 3, pp. 5-26, Jan. 2024, doi: 10.14712/23363177.2023.16.

[220] L. Volante *et al*, "International trends in the implementation of assessment for learning *revisited*: Implications for policy and practice in a post-COVID world," *Policy Futures in Education*, p. 14782103241255855, May 2024, doi: 10.1177/14782103241255855.

[221] I Dewa Ayu Made Meilani Pramesti, "EXPLORING THE BENEFITS OF FORMATIVE ASSESSMENT IN THE CLASSROOM," *esteem*, vol. 6, no. 1, pp. 188-194, Jul. 2024, doi: 10.31851/esteem.v6i1.16142.

[222] K. T. S. Al Harrasi, "Enhancing learner self-monitoring in self-assessment through the use of pedagogical resources," *Cogent Social Sciences*, vol. 10, no. 1, pp. 2334486, Dec. 2024, doi: 10.1080/23311886.2024.2334486.

[223] Department of Civil and Environmental Engineering, The Hong Kong Polytechnic University, Hung Hom, Kowloon, Hong Kong, China, S. Dutta, M. He, Department of Civil and Environmental Engineering, The Hong Kong Polytechnic University, Hung Hom, Kowloon, Hong Kong, China, D. C.W. Tsang, and Department of Civil and Environmental Engineering, The Hong Kong Polytechnic University, Hung Hom, Kowloon, Hong Kong, China, "Reflection and peer assessment to promote self-directed learning in higher education," *J. Edu. Res. Rev.* vol. 11, no. 3, pp. 35-46, Mar. 2023, doi: 10.33495/jerr_v11i3.23.111.

[224] T. Lim, S. Gottipati, and M. L. F. Cheong, "Educational Technologies and Assessment Practices: Evolution and Emerging Research Gaps," in *Advances in Educational Technologies and Instructional Design*, J. Braman, A. Brown, and M. J. Richards, Eds., IGI Global, 2024, pp. 136-172. doi: 10.4018/979-8-3693-1310-7.ch009.
[225] Associate professor of University of economics and pedagogy, Uzbekistan and A. N. Rafiqovna, "THE IMPORTANCE OF PERSONALIZED LEARNING TECHNOLOGIES AND SOME RECOMMENDATIONS," *ajps*, vol. 4, no. 6, pp. 91-93, Jun. 2024, doi: 10.37547/ajps/Volume04Issue06-19.
[226] L.N. Gumilyov Eurasian National University, M. P. Asylbekova, T. N. Otarova, D. C. Yelkin, M.Kh. Dulaty Taraz Regional University, and Yeditepe University, "The importance of transversal skills in higher education curricula and inthe labor market," *BULLETIN of the L.N. Gumilyov Eurasian National University. PEDAGOGY. PSYCHOLOGY. SOCIOLOGY Series*, vol. 142, no. 1, pp. 178-193, 2023, doi: 10.32523/2616-6895-2023-142-1-178-193.
[227] J. Perez Castro, "Pedagogía inclusiva y evaluación de los aprendizajes, una relación compleja," *RDE*, vol. 16, no. 38, p. e16835, Mar. 2024, doi: 10.28998/2175-6600.2024v16n38pe16835.
[228] G. K. Joseph, "BRIDGING CULTURES FOSTERING INCLUSIVE ASSESSMENT OF 21ST CENTURY SKILLS," in *21st Century Teaching and Learning in Classrooms*, First, Sr. G. K Joseph, Prof. (Dr.) K. Y. Benedict, Mrs. S. P K, and Mrs. U. P, Eds., Iterative International Publishers, Selfypage Developers Pvt Ltd, 2024, pp. 1-9. doi: 10.58532/nbennurctch1.
[229] F. X. Pedro and A. C. Teixeira, "The Impact of Accelerated Digital Transformation on Educational Institutions:," in *Advances in Educational Technologies and Instructional Design*, S. M. C. Loureiro and J. Guerreiro, Eds., IGI Global, 2021, pp. 1-26. doi: 10.4018/978-1-7998-6963-4.ch001.
[230] A. Singh, "Digital Transformation in Education: Customary to Digital Education," in *Evolution of Digitized Societies Through Advanced Technologies*, A. Choudhury, T. P. Singh, A. Biswas, and M. Anand,

Eds. in Advanced Technologies and Societal Change. Singapore: Springer Nature Singapore, 2022, pp. 19-32. doi: 10.1007/978-981-19-2984-7_3.

[231] K. Becker, "Integrating a New Framework for Inclusive Evaluation: EPIC-SCREAM," *PAAC*, Oct. 2022, doi: 10.21900/j.alise.2022.1032.

[232] M. A. S. Khasawneh and Y. J. A. Khasawneh, "Achieving Assessment Equity and Fairness: Identifying and Eliminating Bias in Assessment Tools and Practices," Jun. 09, 2023, *Social Sciences*. doi: 10.20944/preprints202306.0730.v1.

[233] Dr. A. B. Tripathy, Dr. B. C. Swain, and Mrs. S. Mishra, "Environmental Sustainability For A Sustainable Future And Role Of Education (In Climate Change Perspectives)," *eatp*, May 2024, doi: 10.53555/kuey.v30i5.5952.

[234] A. R. Hendrada Putri, A. Usman, and H. M. Fashiha, "Development of SESD (Science Education for Sustainable Development) based on Student Worksheet 'Climate Action' Social Science Content to Construct Critical Thinking Skills of Elementary School Students," *Int J Res Rev*, vol. 11, no. 6, pp. 683-691, Jun. 2024, doi: 10.52403/ijrr.20240674.

[235] F. Mrisse, N. Chafiq, and M. Talbi, "Transitioning to Hybrid Assessment: Reflections on Academic Assessment Practices Post-COVID-19," Apr. 08, 2024. doi: 10.32388/MD9JHJ.

[236] C. Hamzaoui, "Overcoming Online Assessment Challenges in Time of a New Normal: Case Study of Belhadj Bouchaib University," *JLT*, vol. 2, no. 2, pp. 134-147, Mar. 2024, doi: 10.70204/jlt.v2i2.251.

[237] I. Karakaya and U. Öç, "Assessment 21st Century Skills: Tools and Methods Used," in *Advances in Educational Technologies and Instructional Design*, E. Yünkül and A. M. Güneş, Eds., IGI Global, 2024, pp. 149-178. doi: 10.4018/979-8-3693-8130-4.ch007.

[238] L. Collins and J. David, "Reflections on Assessment for Development," in *Talent Assessment*, 1st ed, T. Kantrowitz, D. H. Reynolds, and J. Scott, Eds, Oxford University PressNew York, 2023, pp. 328-346. doi: 10.1093/oso/9780197611050.003.0021.

[239] A. Mendonça, K. Freire, and V. Silva, "Continuing training of teachers and pedagogical practices: relationship with knowledge:

Formação continuada de professores e práticas pedagógicas: relação com o saber," *CLIUM*, vol. 23, no. 3, pp. 105-118, Mar. 2023, doi: 10.53660/CLM-853-23B13.

[240] I. Zhorova, O. Kokhanovska, O. Khudenko, N. Osypova, and O. Kuzminska, "Teachers' training for the use of digital tools of the formative assessment in the implementation of the concept of the New Ukrainian School," *Educ. Technol. Q.*, vol. 2022, no. 1, pp. 56-72, Feb. 2022, doi: 10.55056/etq.11.

[241] G. Levitt and S. Grubaugh, "Teacher-centered or Student-centered Teaching Methods and Stu-dent Outcomes in Secondary Schools: Lecture/Discussion and Pro-ject-based Learning/Inquiry Pros and Cons," *JETM*, vol. 1, no. 2, Jun. 2023, doi: 10.59652/jetm.v1i2.16.

[242] F. Yoshida, G. J. Conti, T. Yamauchi, and M. Kawanishi, "Learner-Centeredness vs. Teacher-Centeredness: How Are They Different?," *JEL*, vol. 12, no. 5, p. 1, Jun. 2023, doi: 10.5539/jel.v12n5p1.

[243] Paul Kwame Butakor, "EXPLORING THE EFFECTIVENESS OF ICT TOOLS FOR ONLINE TEACHING, LEARNING AND ASSESSMENT AMONG PRE-SERVICE TEACHERS FROM A GHANAIAN UNIVERSITY," *RS Global - IJITSS*, no. 2(42), May 2024, doi: 10.31435/rsglobal_ijitss/30062024/8162.

[244] A.-L. Cirneanu and C.-E. Moldoveanu, "Use of Digital Technology in Integrated Mathematics Education," *ASI*, vol. 7, no. 4, p. 66, Jul. 2024, doi: 10.3390/asi7040066.

[245] J. Willis, J. Arnold, and C. DeLuca, "Accessibility in assessment for learning: sharing criteria for success," *Front. Educ.* vol. 8, pp. 1170454, May 2023, doi: 10.3389/feduc.2023.1170454.

[246] T. S. Weiss, G. J. Whitman, D. L. Lam, C. M. Straus, and D. S. Sarkany, "A Step-by-Step Approach Addressing Resistance to Appropriately Delivered Constructive Feedback," *Academic Radiology*, vol. 30, no. 12, pp. 3104-3108, Dec. 2023, doi: 10.1016/j.acra.2023.07.012.

[247] A. Lugg, C. Lang, J. Weller, and N. Carr, "Collaboration in a Context of Accountability: Cultural Change in Teacher Educator Practice Across University Boundaries," in *Teaching Performance Assessments as a Cultural Disruptor in Initial Teacher Education*, C. Wyatt-Smith, L. Adie, and J. Nuttall, Eds. in Teacher Education,

Learning Innovation and Accountability. Singapore: Springer Singapore, 2021, pp. 95-114. doi: 10.1007/978-981-16-3705-6_6.

[248] A. Sewell, "Interprofessional Collaboration," in *Diverse Voices in Educational Practice*, 1st ed., London: Routledge, 2022, pp. 64-82. doi: 10.4324/9781003165842-4.

[249] J. Madsen and J. A. Luévanos, "Strategies for Creating Inclusive Schools," *Qeios*, Apr. 2024, doi: 10.32388/P3RQ8K.

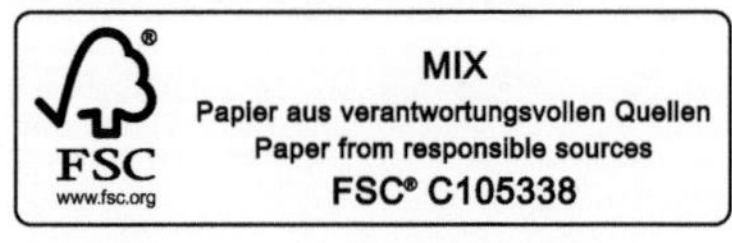

Printed by Books on Demand GmbH, Norderstedt / Germany